ABOUT FACE

*

ABOUT FACE

An Hour a Week to Radiant Skin and Flawless Make-Up

JEFFREY BRUCE

and

SHERRY SUIB COHEN

WITH PHOTOGRAPHS BY MARC RABOY
HAIR STYLES BY STEPHAN PIETRO

G. P. PUTNAM'S SONS * NEW YORK

Library of Congress Cataloging in Publication Data

Bruce, Jeffrey.
About face

Includes index.
1. Beauty, Personal.   2. Face—Care and hygiene.   3. Skin—Care and hygiene.   4. Cosmetics.
I. Cohen, Sherry Suib.   II. Title.
RA778.B915   1983   646.7′26   83-13724
ISBN 0-399-12916-2

Designed by Helen Barrow

PRINTED IN THE UNITED STATES OF AMERICA

* *We're very grateful* . . .

To Diane Reverand, our editor, who gave birth to Daniel and this book in the same nine months. The book took more labor.

To Phyllis Grann, our publisher, for her warmth, her suggestions and for being a good sport.

To Connie Clausen, agent extraordinaire. She tempers pellucid honesty with great good humor.

To our families: Mildred and Edward Hirsch, Lee and Lou Bialick, Stefanie Turnbull, Jane and David Suib, Lee, Larry, Jennifer and Adam Cohen, who are connoisseurs of beauty—inside and out.

To Wayne Brazier for his thoughtful, intelligent insight.

To the stellar women who lent their fabulous faces to our book.

To Teri Seidman—she knows why.

We owe a great debt to two consummate beauty professionals for their collaboration in *About Face*.

MARC RABOY, international celebrity photographer who is represented in almost every major American magazine, *Newsweek, Town and Country, Mademoiselle, Glamour, Gentleman's Quarterly,* and *Interview* being just a few. His clients are world famous and fortunate.

STEPHAN PIETRO, the talented hair designer for many Broadway shows, including *Crimes of the Heart* and *42nd Street,* whose work can be regularly spotted in the national magazines.

JENNY YIP and DAVID HUGHES are the fine artists whose original drawings are graphic explanations. David's work can be found on pages 66–67. All the other illustrations are Jenny's.

7

✳ Contents

PAGE

11 *Prologue*

15 **1. The Bad News**

16 PRODUCT RIP-OFFS: *The Big-Sport Ploy* ✳ *"Holy Cow, It's a Miracle" Creams* ✳ *The "Buy My Whole System" Strategy* ✳ *Department Store Pundits* ✳ *The Soft Soap Strategy*

19 HOAXES: *Do-Everything Products* ✳ *God-Knows-What's-In-Them Products* ✳ *A-Rose-by-Any-Other-Name Products* ✳ *Overpriced Miracle Products*

21 ARROGANT EXPERTS: *Medical Doctors* ✳ *"Beauty Doctors"* ✳ *"Civilian Doctors"*

23 TRAPS OF THE TRADE: *Kitchen Cosmetics* ✳ *Facial Exercises and Massage* ✳ *Yo-Yo Dieting* ✳ *Wrinkle Creams* ✳ *Hormone Hoopla* ✳ *Herpes Havens* ✳ *The pH Balance*

27 CHEAP IS CHEAP—THERE'S NO WAY AROUND IT

31 **2. Saving Face: Skin Care and Maintenance**

31 BLACKHEADS, WHITEHEADS AND ZITS

32 THE SKIN-CARE TWO-STEP: *Step 1: The Night Moves* ✳ *Step 2: The Maintenance Moves* ✳ *Blackhead Emergency Fixes* ✳ *What Happens Next?*

40 THE SKIN YOU'RE IN: *What's Your Skin Type?* ✳ *The Checkpoint Changes of Your Skin* ✳ *Skin Savers* ✳ *Troubletimes* ✳ *The Sun: Friend or Foe?* ✳ *You Are What You Eat—You Look It, Too!* ✳ *Annoyances, Embarrassments, Protuberances and Other Skin-Uglies* ✳ *Sensitive Skin, Allergic Skin*

55 *3. Facing Front: Makeup*

56   *All the Makeup Products You Ever Need* ✳ *Morning Premakeup
        Routine*

60   *THE JEFFREY BRUCE MAKEUP: Makeup—Step by Step* ✳ *Tips
        and Tricks* ✳ *Freebies*

78   *THE BIGGEST MISTAKES: WHICH ONES DO YOU MAKE?*
        ✳ *Nine Big Mistakes* ✳ *Let There Be Light*

83   *INVENT YOURSELF!: Invent Your Eyes* ✳ *Invent Your Nose*
        ✳ *Invent Your Facial Bones* ✳ *Invent a Chinline* ✳ *Invent Your
        Eyebrows*

93   *THE SIMPLEST GUIDE IN THE WORLD TO YOUR BEST
        COLORS: Sallow or Pink–White Skin* ✳ *Ruddy Skin*
        ✳ *Olive–Mediterranean Skin* ✳ *General Color Strategies* ✳ *Eye
        Shadow Color Combos*

98   *THE VERSATILITY OF MAKEUP: The Touch-Up Freshener*
        ✳ *The "Natural" Beauties*

105 *4. The Makeovers*

106   *THE EYES* ✳ *CHEEKBONES—OR LACK OF THEM* ✳ *THE
        NOSE* ✳ *THE MOUTH* ✳ *CHINS AND JAWLINES* ✳ *IN LIVING
        COLOR: THE MAKEOVERS EXPLAINED* ✳ *SKIN* ✳ *HALF
        FACES*

123 *5. Special People, Special Places*

123   *AN UNDER-EIGHTEEN SKIN CARE AND MAKEUP GUIDE:
        Makeup for Minors: Ten Steps to Dynamite!*

129   *BEST FACE FORWARD: OVER FORTY: Clean Up Your Act!*
        ✳ *Grown-Up Beauty*

134   *SKIN CARE AND MAKEUP FOR THE BIG WOMAN: First, Skin
        Care* ✳ *Now, Makeup*

137   *BLACK BEAUTY AND SKIN CARE: Skin Care for the Black
        Woman* ✳ *Makeup*

143   *HELLO PREGNANCY: GOODBYE (FOR A WHILE) GREAT SKIN*

144   *MAKEUP FOR SPECIAL TIMES: Beauty in the Bed* ✳ *Beauty on the
        Beach* ✳ *Beauty and the Blues* ✳ *Beauty for the Blurry-Eyed*

147 *6. Cosmetic Facial Surgery: How to Avoid the Glazed Ham Look*

Eyelid Surgery * *Chin and Neck Surgery* * *The Face-Lift* * *Peel It Off?* * *Dermabrasion* * *Electrocautery* * *The Collagen Connection* * *Seven Questions Most Often Asked About Cosmetic Surgery* * *The Last Word*

153 *Epilogue*

155 *Index*

A NOTE TO THE READER

The opinions expressed in this book are just that—opinions. My opinions. They are not statements of irrefutable fact. When I speak of specific products, I am giving you my impressions of them only. You may think differently, as is your absolute right.

Prologue

I AM a makeup and skin-care artist. I love my work. Why? Picture the following scene that occurred last week: as soon as it happened I was determined to begin my book with it.

An intelligent woman enters my studio. She has been recommended by a client who is in the theater, but she herself has nothing to do with show business. She's a lawyer, as it happens; an enormously successful, articulate advocate. What's more, I subsequently hear, she has had great personal success. Married for twenty-five years to a man who adores her, she has two children who not only love but admire their terrific mother.

She sits slumped over in my chair, making clever and self-deprecating remarks. She's not wearing a drop of makeup; her hair is obviously clean but limp and shapeless.

"Can you fix this face?" she asks. "Consider it your greatest challenge . . . I'm not just another pretty face. . . ." And so on. She makes a lot of jokes. She's very clever.

I start to work; she doesn't stop talking, laughing. I clean her face, apply a freshener, a base, begin to work on sculpting bones with contour. As I work, she begins to quiet. I almost feel an imperceptible relaxation of her facial muscles as she starts to change from plain to absolutely pretty. I add color, blusher. She's begun to sit straighter in her chair. I'm not surprised. It always happens.

When I get to her eyes, she hasn't made a joke or said a word for five minutes. She's just watching herself grow pretty—maybe for the first time in her adult life. The first eye shadow goes on. The second. Her eyes have come alive. By God, they're not dull brown, they're *taupe*, with glistening, wonderful specks of gold in them. Two more shadows, the eyeliner, the mascara. The lady is breathtaking.

And then it happens. It always does. She looks at herself in the mirror, this new sensual creature, and *she sucks in her cheeks.* It's an almost universal reaction. When a woman looks into a mirror, feeling newly sophisticated, newly wonderful, she sucks in her cheeks, sits up tall in her chair and gives off an aura of "Well, look at that. I'm sensational!"

I finish my work. The lawyer sits there, very quietly. She looks at herself from many angles.

Then she looks at me. "Thanks," she says. No jokes, no wisecracks, no slumping in the chair. "I didn't know anyone could do this. I feel very . . . good-looking," she says. "Pretty" is not a word in her vocabulary, when she speaks of herself. It will be.

As I said before, I love my work. I love to watch the transformation happen. It gives me, I must admit, a certain kind of power—a power to make people change.

Never knock makeup. You can be the most loved, the busiest, the most creative person in the world; and if you don't feel pretty, there's something missing. It's not enough to have your friends and family love you for yourself, although that surely helps. It's soul-satisfying to know you look smashing. And if that's vanity, well then, vanity is a useful thing. Oh, sure, inner beauty, love of life, goodness all count very much. But since almost every woman can also look wonderful, why not have that too? It's not too much to ask. It doesn't take very much time or money. It makes you walk tall. It really does. I can show you how to do it.

But before I do, I want to tell you that although beauty is my business, everything in the business is far from beautiful. Sometimes it gets downright sordid among all these sweet-smelling jars. It is quite possible, for instance, that the same newly-pretty lawyer I just described will come back to me next week absolutely hooked on a "scientific" claim, a cleverly phrased implication that if she plunks down three hundred dollars of her last hard-earned legal fee for Dr. Scientific's DewYouth Beauty Regimen, she will become irresistibly, heartstoppingly young, forever. It doesn't matter how savvy or sophisticated she is, claims like that can easily sweep her off her feet. But it won't come true. It's one more lie from a fat-cat, gleeful cosmetic company.

This enrages me, and that's why, for a long time, I've wanted to write this book. Professional muckrakers have alluded to the various myths (they range from "the most expensive is the best" to "the cheapest is the best") but I don't think anyone *within* the beauty business has ever really exposed the nefarious tricks of the trade. I propose to do just that.

I also want to write a book that simply, honestly tells women how to be their most beautiful. Beauty, you see, the kind that's possible with cosmetics, has nothing to do with "primary color identities," "mystical auras," or "summer and winter personalities"—some of the more offensive hype I've been seeing lately. It has everything to do with learning how to put what creams and what colors on what places. It has everything to do with a clean face. All else is witless nonsense.

This book is also about choice. I tell you that I have my own line of cosmetics that is carefully created by my own chemists according to my own very specific instructions; and I think it's a wonderful, quality, honest line. But there are many other fine cosmetics, and as this book progresses, I'll mention some that I think have been consistently reliable. I can't *understand* why every makeup artist who values integrity doesn't do exactly that. But can you imagine Adrien Arpel telling you to try Max Factor? It's so silly. How can you be a credible authority if you only push your own line, if you don't admit that your product is not unique in all the world? The only way to be an intelligent cosmetics consumer is to test, reject, select. I'd love it if you decide that Jeffrey Bruce Cosmetics are the only ones that make you look fantastic. But you won't. And they're not.

So, here's this long-thought-out book's promise:

* It will tell you what's pure hype and chicanery in this business.
* It will give you choices.
* It will teach you how to create absolutely wonderful skin.
* It will teach you how to be your most beautiful self—via makeup.
* It will tell the truth.

But first, the bad news . . .

1 *

The Bad News

"MY COUNTRY, right or wrong," goes the chauvinistic statement, implying fanatical belief in something because it belongs to you. Well, that may be all very right for countries, but I can't buy it for professions. The beauty business is mine and it has been good to me, and there is much that is original and delightful and psyche-supporting in it; but it is also a business where there is so much wrong that it's embarrassing. "Spend all you have for loveliness. Buy it and never count the cost," wrote poet Sara Teasdale, and she knew what she was talking about because millions of people who can little afford that philosophy still spend many billions of dollars on lipstick and rouge and mauve eye shadow. Class, intellect, age, profession, geography and marital status are all transcended when you're selling beauty. People who consider themselves beyond the frivolity of foundation come running and pushing to your door when you tell them you'll show them how to make their eyes look larger. Women and men who *hate* themselves for caring so much care nevertheless. That makes us easy dupes for those who are very good at selling dreams.

Now, there's nothing wrong with buying dreams if the dream has a hope of coming true. Dream it enough, and the reality comes to echo the dream. You can rewrite the future if you're happy about the way you look, and don't discount the fun you have in playing with your face's possibilities. Applying makeup is a sensual, pleasurable activity, and if you buy honest products and advice you're getting full value.

But, as in every field, there are charlatans at work. Not satisfied with the enormous profits that can come from offering legitimate products and legitimate advice, the stuff of *good* dreams, the giants of the cosmetics industry have created a nightmare of silliness. Along with the workable products and advice, consumers have been sold perhaps the world's most expensive "face job" from corporate wordsmiths who are very good at doling out high-price delusions. Women are sold "cell renewal" even though they know better. Fortunes can be made if you are clever enough to think of twelve ways to say pink . . . and sell the same color to the same person twelve different times. Just because you are buying, the industry is selling. Along with the legitimate, too many in the business are selling pure hype and tricks that can't work—calling it glamour, calling it truth.

I believe in cosmetics, in makeup. That's why it distresses me when I see the industry lying, pulling punches, pushing the mediocre. Elaborate, national pushes to get a consumer to change lipstick colors as often as she changes her underwear have *got* to backfire and create distrust. We have such a good thing in the beauty business—teaching and helping people to look wonderful—why do we have to spoil it all by overkill? The answer, I suppose, is greed. In order to make more money, too many companies imply they have eternal youth, sex and popularity to sell instead of just plain old looking good.

I'm not interested in rocking the cosmetics industry. What I am interested in is preserving the dignity and integrity of my profession. It's a self-serving interest, I must admit. It's easier to defend and live with truth. Therefore, what follows in this chapter are some of the more nefarious tricks of the trade—the ones that *don't* do you any good.

PRODUCT RIP-OFFS

The Big-Sport Ploy

Every woman has received those smelly little packets from her favorite department store, which promise "free" merchandise if she makes a purchase. Now, your mother told you that nothing is free, and she was right. What you are getting in those "free" gifts are the back supplies and the mistakes of the company making you the offer. Things that didn't sell because they're not terrific. Orange lipsticks, pistachio eye shadows, aqua lip liners—colors that clash and shriek instead of complement. Those are your prizes, your "free gift with purchase."

Industry does not waste merchandise it can sell, and much of the time, these gifts are the surplus the company is trying to unload because they're merchandising washouts. Estēe Lauder started the idea when she was involved in the great competition with Revlon and it caught on like hotcakes—the old something-for-nothing tactic. It's true that sometimes you're even offered a "hot" item as a gift along with purchase. Rest assured, in this case the amount you receive is probably so infinitesimal as to be practically useless in a fair trial of the product. The company feels that the customer might just come back for a bigger investment in a product she's been given a whiff of. Often a company will up the price of a product, give you a "gift" of a free sample, and more than make back its cost by the price increase.

Sometimes the Big-Sport Ploy backfires and costs the company more than it planned. So the company recoups its losses. How, you ask? By an almost unbelievable bit of customer-patronizing that actually works. (I cannot fathom why for the life of me.) The magicians at customer-manipulation figured out that they can even *charge* for a "gift" and still have the customer make a purchase for the privilege of buying the gift. The ads tell you that if you make any purchase you will be "allowed" to buy this other product for "only $10.95." Thanks, but no thanks.

Other companies ignore the fact that they're supposed to be makeup experts and offer you absolute irrelevancies as bait. Lauren gives luggage away, Gloria Vanderbilt, Aramis and others dabble in umbrellas, Lancôme pushes handbags. What's more, this type of gift serves another purpose for the company—that of free advertising, since its name is plastered all over your "gift." Now what has this to do with concern and respect for or true interest in a consumer's face? Nothing, I suggest.

"Holy Cow, It's a Miracle" Creams

Christine Valmy touts a chicken placenta masque for very dry skin at $54.30. Looking for more exotica? Livia Sylva of the New York Clinique de Beauté swears by shark oil. The Klisar Skin Care Center in New York loves seaweed. Ilona of Hungary whips up quail egg omelets for your face. Polly Bergen preferred turtles: Her miracle cream suggested that turtle oil will do the trick for you—it didn't. Looking for exotic oil extracts? Jōvan pushes minks. Someone else touts bees' jelly.

There are all kinds of exotica in "miracle creams" which add nothing to the efficacy of a product, and everything to its value to the copywriters. Federal law does not state that cosmetics have to be effective, only reasonably safe, therefore the copywriters get away with murder.

Comes the inevitable question to Jeffrey Bruce: "How come you tout *aloe* as the miracle ingredient in *your* products? Isn't it the same thing?" It isn't. For centuries aloe has been a healing agent for *human beings,* not for bees, chickens or turtles. Just last week Stephan Pietro, who is responsible for the hair styles in this book, gouged his face terribly while horseback riding during his vacation on a tropical island. A local person immediately suggested juice from the aloe plant, which grows abundantly in that area. He lathered himself with the aloe liquid and the wound was gone in six days without leaving a scar. Burns respond extraordinarily to aloe. It heals, it nourishes, and, because it has a high volume of water, it moisturizes. It is not a fad, not a fly-by-night ad-writer's campaign—it is a centuries-old skin balm. I did not invent it.

The "Buy My Whole System" Strategy

There are other types of product rip-offs, in my opinion, and one of the worst is any system that says you have to use it exclusively—or else smother in pimples. The companies which push these "systems" usually deal with gimmicks that are so modern, so wise and so fail-proof, you wouldn't dare pit your wisdom against, say, a computer that analyzes skin problems and prescribes cosmetics to cure them.

One of these systems is the Erno Laszlo Skincare System. Laszlo, a Hungarian dermatologist, devised a ritual that proved irresistible to many women, who learned that they must follow his regimen to the letter, use *only* his products and, to have the privilege of doing so, must join the Erno Laszlo Institute and be a "member," which costs about $250. Just anyone can't buy Laszlo products; you have to fill out a long questionnaire called a Dermatological Review and pay for the honor of being "Laszloed." (Making it hard is a brilliant marketing device.) You have to present a membership card to buy a product: that appeals to the most consummate of snobs who love exclusive practices. Their records, they are told, are sent to the Erno Laszlo Institute.

"The skin speaks to me in Hungarian," the great Doctor Laszlo has said.

And what's the basis of the "finest skincare system in the world"? It's simply washing with Sea Mud Soap (whatever that is, which sells for an astronomical fifteen dollars per bar of soap, would you believe ? !).

This is not to say that I disapprove of all Laszlo products. I don't, and surely there are many good things to say about some of them. What I strongly object to is the *system* of seducing the consumer, the hype and the hoopla that goes along with the product. It's patronizing.

The "Buy My Whole System" strategy, once marketed for just the very rich, has now filtered down to middle and lower income consumers who are treated to similar lines in the "personalized" door-to-door campaigns of companies like Avon and Mary Kay. The "trained" specialists in these companies try to give the illusion that their individualized attention is what's best for you, and that to buy the whole line of products makes *scientific* sense. This new door-to-door, at-home cosmetic campaign often robs the consumer of the chance to compare prices as she could in a department store, and she often ends up spending far more on her "bargain" line than she would in the store. You *never* have to buy a whole line to insure uniformity of results.

And, while I'm on the subject, anyone who would buy a cosmetics beauty book from a company which touts only its own line deserves what she gets : an expensive advertisement.

Department Store Pundits

Another way to get ripped off with certain products is to buy— lock, stock and barrel— the advice of the salesperson (often dressed in a convincing doctor's smock) selling that product. What you are really doing is taking the advice of someone who was probably selling pantyhose on another floor last week, and

is interested in commissions and sales—not your skin purity or even, believe it or not, your beauty. The Estēe Lauder, Revlon, Germaine Monteil or Clinique salesperson is *not* your best friend. Often, she is not even very knowledgeable about the product she's pushing.

The Soft Soap Strategy

Sure, soap cleans. It cleans because it's such a good degreaser, but in the process it can actually degrease *you* and lower your natural facial oil content by as much as one-third. Soap is not your friend : I hate to see anyone over age ten use soap on her face. But you use *special* soaps you say ? Let's take a look at these special soaps.

MOISTURIZING SOAPS   First of all, they're not chock full of moisture (which is water) but oil. And they're pure hype because the excess of fatty oils (the moisturizing part) gets washed off for the most part, and goes down the drain along with the rinse water. If any should remain, it sits on top of the skin as a thin coat of oil, insidiously clogging your pores. They may be okay for the body with its less sensitive skin, but I can't think of a good thing to say about moisturizing soaps used on the face. Whether your skin is dry or not, the fatty acids will almost surely irritate it.

MEDICATED SOAPS   These are generally useless because the medication usually goes down the drain the moment you rinse. Antibacterial soaps have also been known to kill the skin's natural bacteria, which give it immunity from infection.

Black women with troubled complexions ought to avoid medicated soaps containing resorcinol which can darken skin and create blotches.

<u>PERFUMED SOAPS</u> They're the worst skin irritants I can think of. These include all the most common supermarket soaps as well as the higher priced brands. They're also detergent soaps which means they lather well but are very irritating to skin.

<u>DEODORANT SOAPS</u> These products contain chemicals that can be irritating if all of the deodorant part isn't flushed away with the rinse—which makes it meaningless in the first place.

Soap's not even cheap any more. Why would anyone use it instead of a nice, gentle cleansing cream or lotion? If anyone tells you that soap will moisturize or in other ways be good for your skin, *do not believe it!*

HOAXES

Do-Everything Products

Too often, one sees a product advertised as having a multitude of virtues. It's supposed to take off makeup, put back moisture, close pores, open pores—in short, work magic. Distrust this product. It cannot do all the things it promises. In order for it to be a cleanser, it should be able to open pores to let the dirt out. How can it be an astringent, which closes pores, at the same time? How can it be a moisturizer, which has to be a lot gentler than a cleansing cream? Noxzema Complexion Lotion, touted as having many of the aforementioned properties, is really only a rinse-off cleanser, and because of its watery and thin consistency, I find that it is not even very good at taking makeup off.

Helena Rubinstein puts out an Eye Cream Special that is designed to be used at night *or* under makeup. Can't be both, I say. When makeup is used, the eye should be kept as arid as possible, otherwise the makeup will congeal; coagulate in cracks and lines. Eye cream should be used at night—only. In my opinion, Rubinstein's eye cream is too heavy even for night use; many of my clients have complained that it causes puffiness and swelling. At any rate, because it's rather greasy and heavy, using it under makeup would be a big mistake. Eye creams are not designed for day and night use: it's almost a contradiction in terms.

The new "super-creams," advertised as going farther than moisturizing or stimulating or lubricating, are promoted as age controllers. That's simply not true. Nothing can control age. Creams cannot preserve youth and beauty even if they can improve skin texture. So please be wary of products which promise the moon.

God-Knows-What's-In-Them Products

Consumers must be aware of what their special needs are in order to know if the products they choose are really right for them. It is an advertising hoax, in my judgment, to point a product to a specific age or skin-type group, and then ignore the needs of that group. For example: Bonne Bell products are marketed for very young women. They're supposed to be terrific for teenagers. Why, then, does the Bonne Bell Moisture Lotion have perfume and mineral oil in it which makes it irritating and sticky—the antithesis of what the adolescent skin can use? Teenagers have enough problems without the extra irritation perfumes can supply and the extra oil present in the mineral oil.

Revlon is another manufacturer that has come out with a product supposedly geared for a special group of consumers and has then virtually ignored the needs of that group. In order to tap the black-skin market, they introduced a line called Polished Ambers whose purpose was to do wonderful things for the eyes and skin of the black woman. Well, the cream-on eye shadows were shiningly irridescent golds and browns, in my opinion and in the estimation of impartial research coordinators harsh, unflattering shades, *especially* to black skins. What's more, I have seen the Polished Ambers cream foundation turn grey and green on black women—they are simply not compatible with some black skin.

Ralph Lauren pushes the ''natural'' look in makeup and gears his advertisements to a barely postpubescent mark. His blushers are phosphorescent. A heliotrope eye shadow looks like you stuck a flashlight inside of an eggplant. Not so ''natural,'' after all.

Christine Valmy puts out a product obviously geared for the older woman, Valtone Eye and Neck Creme. The product contains extracts of mint, lavender and lemon, none of which is terrifically soothing to thinner, dryer, aging skin. Many of my clients report the opposite benefit intended; instead of diminishing puffiness under their eyes, it increases puffiness and irritation.

I could go on . . .

A-Rose-by-Any-Other-Name Products

For a long time, I've had a suspicion that many companies put out very similar products marketed under different names, and sell them for varying amounts depending upon the prestige of the company. Revlon, for instance, owns Moon Drops, Etherea, Borghese and Charlie products. Estēe Lauder owns Clinique, Aramis, Prescriptives and the Lauder line. All of these products come from the same parent-owned factory. I can't prove it, but one day I will have my own chemist analyze the different products to see if there are significant differences. Now, there's nothing illegal about this, I suppose, but if they're all basically the same product, it's just another example of pulling the wool over the consumer's eyes.

Overpriced Miracle Products

If they were really miracles, well then, why not? But, barring miracles, *no* product is worth its weight in gold. I happen to believe that you get what you pay for: that bargain cosmetics and skin care products are almost always unreliable. Nevertheless, there's a limit. Too many companies are exploiting the snob-appeal theory, the thinking that says if you make an item very expensive and very exclusive, the person who buys it will feel very expensive and very exclusive. That's the reasoning that (very profitably) went behind putting little initials all over everything. The woman who carried a purse covered with D's was letting people know, not very subtly I'm afraid, that I'm a Woman With a Whole Lot of Money, World! The very high price of the item, rather than its inherent goodness, created its desirability. Writer Kathrin Perutz tells the story of the American woman in Paris who was outraged when Dior created a hat for her in just a few moments and said, ''Voilá! Five hundred dollars, Madame.'' ''Five hundred dollars!'' gasped the woman incredulously. ''Why, it's just a piece of ribbon!'' Dior leaned over, solemnly unraveled the ribbon and handed it to the woman with great ceremony. ''The ribbon, Madame, is free,'' said the famous designer with magnanimity. He knew what the name Dior was worth. And so, with cosmetics also, there are those who pay a fortune an ounce for fancy packaging, fancy names and export duties from fancy countries, even though the creams are no better at all than their more modest counterparts.

If a product is really extraordinary, then a high price is not out of line, but if a product is just mediocre (and only you can judge that), you would be foolish to plunk down a lot of pennies. Beautiful packaging, foreign-sounding names and exotic smells, rather than quality, are what earn the marketing geniuses the really extraordinary salaries they more than deserve.

Look—*hope* is worth a great deal. I'm not telling you that you're a fool to pay an exorbitant amount for a product when there's a *reasonable* chance that hope will turn into reality. To pay for pure hype just because it's very glittery, instead of reasonable hope, does not make sense. Overpriced miracles too often land with dull thuds in your wastepaper basket.

ARROGANT EXPERTS

Medical Doctors

If your skin is not primarily a medical problem you may be making a big mistake by putting it into the hands of a dermatologist. People often worship their doctors, put them on pedestals, never question their judgment. As a result, doctors, in my opinion, began to take on a certain air of arrogance. We believed they could do no wrong and they be-

gan to believe it also. A certain cavalier attitude in many medical people became the norm instead of the exception. If you asked a question, they said, ''Trust me—you wouldn't understand.'' And too many of us relinquished responsibility for our bodies. When things went wrong, and they did, we simply assumed there was no better way to have handled it; after all, it was a *doctor* who told us the way to go.

Now, there are good doctors and there are thoughtless doctors, as in every profession. A thoughtless skin doctor will cause you great needless grief and will waste your money because he or she simply would rather medicate than teach you to cleanse properly, rather operate than spend weeks clearing up the skin with a nonsurgical procedure. Sometimes it's not just thoughtlessness, it's greed. One makes a better living when one keeps a patient dependent upon one's skill.

In the area of skin care, where so much depends on cleanliness habits, it's particularly easy to say to your dermatologist, ''You do it,'' instead of taking on responsibility for your own face. A good skin care and makeup expert has to have many clients because if he or she's really good, he'll teach you how to keep your skin wonderful and how to apply makeup, and then you're finished with each other, except for an occasional appointment. But, if you make going to the expert (doctor or beauty) a way of life, it's an ongoing process. With skin care, that is simply not necessary unless, as I said earlier, you have serious medical problems.

Dermatologists too often prescribe medicated ointments (which invariably create dryness and other problems) instead of prescribing a good home-facial routine. Too often, they dig and scrape and gouge at skin to remove impurities when a simple exfoliating cream and masque will do the same thing *without* creating pitted areas. Medication often inhibits the sebum, keeps it under the skin for a while. That's fine—until it explodes when it hits four or five other pores and yields a cluster of pimples where only one would have existed if the pus or the sebum was forced to the surface with a good facial.

It has become very fashionable for mothers, themselves dermatology addicts, to bring their pubescent daughters and sons to the Great Skin Doctor, where the youngsters are lanced, squeezed, dug at, ultraviolet-rayed and cortisoned instead of being taught to cleanse, pure and simple. What's more, these same parents are told to keep their daughters away from all makeup—no exceptions—if skin purity is desired. What happens is that the young women study with their faces held in their dirty hands and are exposed to extremes of hot and cold weather, without benefit of protection from makeup and moisturizers. Their skins become terrible and are never cured.

The clients who come to me with the *worst* skin are those who have made a practice of running to their skin doctors at the first sign of trouble. I know that's a blanket statement but I'll stand by it. What's more, Sherry, the coauthor of this book, assures me that her attorney husband has many malpractice cases against dermatologists; for instance, doctors who have created facial holes because they were too quick to use a knife instead of a skin cleanser.

So, there it is: if your skin doctor assures you that you cannot live without his or her degree, try it my way first. Clean up your act, get to the root, the dirt root, of your facial blemishes. I fervently believe that skin care experts who are not medical doctors will always pay more attention to causes than to penicillin. If your skin is a medical problem, of course you'll need a medical doctor. But in most cases, an excellent skin care program will do the trick, and a masque beats out medicine every time.

"Beauty Doctors"

Medical doctors aren't the only ones who display holier-than-thou arrogance. Beauty doctors, in the form of hairdressers, makeup and skin care practitioners and fashion designers, are rife with know-it-all mannerisms. Any time a hairdresser ignores your instructions on cutting or not cutting your hair, make sure you never go back. Any time a makeup artist or a fashion expert treats you in a condescending and patronizing manner, make sure you tell him or her how tacky and low-class that behavior is. Always insist on explanations when a new treatment or style is being suggested, and if you spot that "trust me" attitude don't accept it. Snobbishness can be intimidating if you don't realize that a snobbish attitude comes from a person's own insecurity about self-worth. The beauty expert who would have you cowed in subservience is not worth any expense. You have to be crazy to pay for an insult. If your skin-care expert insists on avocado face masks, make sure you are told what avocado really does that's so great (nothing, if you ask me).

"Civilian Doctors"

I call them civilians—the ones who are not in the business. They're your mother, your next-door neighbor, the local columnist. Indeed, some of them have very good ideas and advice . . . sometimes. And many of them don't. Don't believe everything you read: A columnist who writes on political doings in town may one day be assigned to write a piece about skin—without any personal knowledge of skin. Advice from her is created by the amount of research she does on a subject. Sometimes an article is created out of pure imagination.

Advice on anything is as good as the background of the person who's giving the advice. In your Aunt Sadie's case, that's not so good when she tells you that facial steaming over a pot of hot water will clear up your acne. It didn't clear them up for Sadie and it won't for you. Your mother may tell you to lather dollops of cold cream on your face because that's what her mother did for skin care: there's a lot better on the market for you today than the prehistoric cold creams, a mixture of olive oil, wax and water, the first formula for which was published 1900 years ago by a Greek doctor. It was called cold cream because it cooled the skin as the water evaporated. The trouble with the old cold cream, as well as many cleansing creams of today, is that it leaves a great residue of oily film behind on the skin, even after you take it off. Your pores simply never get unplugged from the stuff and using it often produces absolutely dreadful cases of acne.

So, carefully consider the advice of the Civilian Doctors: And before you do anything that may cause damage, do a little research on the subject at the local library or with a well-respected beauty expert. The responsibility for your face is your own, in the final analysis. Face up to that.

TRAPS OF THE TRADE

I suppose every industry has its placebos and its charlatans and, I'm sorry to say, the cosmetics industry has more than its share. The temptation is irresistible because the need is so naked. It's human, not just feminine, to want to make a terrific impression. Tell the truth, now: If you *really* thought there was a good chance you could be more beautiful, more desirable, more lovable, wouldn't you try? Wouldn't you buy almost any pie-in-the-sky idea? The beauty business is founded on the sure bet that people care how they look, no matter how they protest that it's "what's inside that counts." Sure, what's inside counts, but make no mistake: what's outside often paves the way in emotional and professional relationships and success. Although humans are the only species that use artificial means to ornament themselves with beauty, most animals preen their fur, tail feathers or horns in order to decorate themselves in ways they think make them sexually attractive. The difference between women and peacocks, say, is that women (and men) are attracted to changing fads which they believe make them look good while peacocks rely on the same old colors and tail fluffing every season. It's this faddish aspect to cosmetics and skin care that gets women in trouble the most, although to be fair, modern science does come up with something new every now and then that really does work. I suppose the make-believe aspect—buying the possibility of a dream come true—has, at least, psychological benefits. As long as you don't go broke or hurt yourself, gambling on beauty promises is not as bad as most other kinds of gambles.

There are, though, certain Traps of the Trade, certain promises made by "experts," that anger me more than others. These are the promises that can either really harm you or cause you to throw out money without a hope of the promise coming true. I know it, the people making the promises know it and now you'll know it, too. Let's look at the worst of them.

Kitchen Cosmetics

Most of the time, they're garbage. A spate of books is flooding the market these days, telling women that they need go no farther than their refrigerators to find beautiful skin. Unless you want skin that looks like lemon or avocado skin or is as lumpy as yogurt, don't use these foods on your face. First of all, you do *not* save a mint using mint and the like on your face. If you buy any food product for your face and don't use it up almost immediately it will become rancid very quickly. Which is why cosmetics contain preservatives. In order to be economically intelligent, a cosmetic ought to have a shelf-life that's longer than a couple of days. The eighty-nine cents you spend three or four times weekly on an avocado masque is too much money—that's assuming the avocado even works, which it doesn't.

The current popularity of kitchen cosmetics arises from the notion that natural products put together from berries, herbs, fruits and milk products are better for your skin than non-natural products. Wrong. Do you realize how easy it is to contaminate pores with spoiled products which may not even looked spoiled? There's nothing like a rotten cucumber to promote acne. Remember that the word *natural* doesn't have to be synonymous with *good*. Poison ivy comes from a natural plant. Skin cancer is caused by the natural sun. Certain diseases are caused by natural bacteria. A natural product can do you in. Most vitamins and nutrients can't be absorbed by the skin, but must be broken down by the digestive tract to do you any good. And a mango face mush can get you very moldy.

Originally, cosmetics were made from natural ingredients because science had not yet come up with anything else. Natural has now progressed to synthetic (it's not a dirty word) ingredients which give you far greater efficacy, choice in colors, shelf life and life on the skin. The fact is that you can easily get the few (and I mean few) organic properties that *mean* something in a safer form in laboratory-produced cosmetics. If you were to put natural aloe directly on the skin it would be far too strong. A chemist can include it in a synthetic product in just the right amount. Reduced to dry particles, the natural ingredients are also not susceptible to oxidation and air contamination. Aside from the fact that kitchen cosmetics don't really save you money in the long run and can contaminate your skin, here's what the more popular "natural" products can really do to you.

APRICOTS AND PEACHES   They do as little for the skin as they do to cure cancer.

AVOCADOS   They're practically pure oil, and used on any skin, dry or oily, can clog pores faster than Wesson. Ditto mayonnaise.

EGGS   No one has ever proved that eggs do anything at all for the skin (or hair, either, for that matter). Do you like to smell eggy?

LEMONS   There's a lot of acid in lemons, and using the pure product can create surface dryness and irritations faster than a desert sandstorm. For that reason, the lemon smell you get in most commercially produced cosmetics is not lemon at all, but a substance with almost no acid in it. It's added to make the cosmetic pleasing to the consumer's nose and for no other reason. The same goes for limes and grapefruits. My colleague, Adrien Arpel, suggests a Fruit Punch Facial made up from pure yogurt, lemon juice, lime juice and grapefruit juice. It is my opinion that you ought to drink the thing but never put it on your face!

PINEAPPLES These fruits have strong fermenting qualities that digest dead cells. Also, in my experience, live ones.

STRAWBERRIES More people get allergic reactions from strawberries than penicillin.

YOGURT It is surely nourishing when eaten but doesn't do a single thing on your face, except feel cool. A wet rag will be less sticky and expensive and accomplish the same purpose.

GLYCERINE AND LANOLIN PRODUCTS In dry climates or rooms, glycerine works in total opposition to the concept of moisturizing: it draws water *from* the skin. Only use a product with glycerine in a very humid climate where it will draw moisture from the air. Lanolins in products are also potential problems because lanolins are allergens, substances that can cause allergies.

HEALTH STORE STUFF If you put shark oil, almond or wheat germ oil, bees' royal jelly, squalene, jojoba oil or allantoin on your face you get what you deserve: pimples. Oil products clog and do not moisturize. Only water products moisturize.

"NATURAL" PRODUCTS Beware the pretty, colorful bottles of "natural cosmetics" which might make you sneeze faster than most polluted cosmetics you buy in Bloomingdale's. Read the labels on natural cosmetics: There is no United States ruling on using the word "natural" on labels, and what's natural to the health food store can be conjunctivitis to you.

Facial Exercises and Massage

Doing facial exercises is one of the industry's biggest traps. Manipulating your facial muscles and grimacing in a hundred horrible ways can do nothing good for your skin: All it can do is stretch the skin tissue and cause facial sag in awesome proportions. A very gentle facial massage can feel good, but vigorous massage or exercises can actually break down the connective tissue at the base of the skin and, Hello wrinkles and hang! Dr. Peter Linden, a New York plastic surgeon, says that the many, many facial muscles don't get any benefit from the hours of exercises your faddish "aesthetician" has prescribed and demonstrated at great cost to you. And all you'll ever get is a headache from your chinstrap and your wrinkle-removing headband.

Yo-Yo Dieting

Along with the physical fitness craze has come a plethora of diets. Some of them are worse than torture and others are bearable. At last count, we had about seventy-two thousand to choose from including: the Scarsdale Diet, the Southampton Diet, the Beverly Hills Diet, the Rockefeller Diet, the Last Chance Diet, the Eat All You Want Diet, the Drinking Man's Diet, the Ice Cream Diet, the Starch Blockers' Diet, the Mayo Clinic Diet—I could go on. Now, every reasonable person knows that in the end the only way to lose weight is to stop eating, or at least to stop eating so much. And I don't mean for a week or a month. You must modify your eating habits so you don't make a pattern of gaining and losing. The norm must be a steady eating mode with an occasional binge to preserve your sanity and humanity: not the other way around. If you gain and lose and gain and lose again, you are subjecting yourself to more arterial fat-clogging than if your weight stays consistently high. Moreover, yo-yo diets give you more wrinkles and sagging skin than a basset hound. If you are interested in firm and taut skin you will not opt for a life of binge and diet. It is better for your skin, and for your health, to stay plump. Do not buy another diet book; you have enough already. Just decide to eat a *little* of everything and stay on an even keel.

Wrinkle Creams

Don't spend another dime on any product that promises to remove wrinkles. That's the biggest hype, the biggest trap of all. *Nothing* removes wrinkles. There are some products which cleanse and exfoliate your skin very well and when the dead skin cells and the dirt are removed from the facial lines the wrinkles may *seem* ~~to~~ be smoothed out. That's a good in itself, of course, but the wrinkles have not been removed.

Masques can force your face to relax because it's hard to crinkle up under a masque. When the masque is removed the face does *seem* less lined because it's relaxed, but the wrinkles have not been removed. Ever since Nefertiti wrinkle creams have been pushed. The first ones included sugar and barley water paste, egg white and gelatin which all dry on the face as a masque does and make you look, temporarily, less wrinkled. Take the masque off—and you're back to reality.

The words you have to watch for are many and varied, but they're all the best euphemisms the cosmetic companies have for trapping you with the promise of wrinkle-free skin. When Clinique says that its 7th-day Scrub Cream is a "De-Aging Expert," Germaine Monteil says it has a "Super Moist Line-Stop Creme Concentrate," Stendhal says its eye masque will "reduce tiny wrinkles," Estēe Lauder says she has a "Swiss Age-Controlling Cream"—they're trying to tell you that their products make wrinkles vanish, make age go away. Don't believe it. Skin creams *can* clean, moisturize, soften. They can slow the lines from coming. They can mute the lines already there so they don't look as deep. But if you're destined to get wrinkles, bags, sags at an early age, you will. Your genes, your grandmother, has decreed it.

Hormone Hoopla

Although hormones taken by pill or injection do have very real effects (sometimes beneficial, sometimes not) on menopausal women, hormone creams are thought by most experts to be useless. Claims that they increase elasticity, restore the youthful appearance of the skin, strengthen a thinning epidermis brought on by years and aid the skin in water retention are spurious. What they can do is promote a temporary swelling of the skin which, in effect, plumps out the wrinkles and makes them less noticeable for a while, but the risks of fooling around with hormones are not worth this fleeting benefit. Creams that contain estrogen or progesterone can have dangerous side effects that may not even show up for a while. What's more, hormone creams often increase the growth of facial hair, an effect not welcomed by too many women.

Placenta masques and extracts rely on hormones. You'll pay extravagantly for the doubtful benefits, at least fifty dollars for a minuscule amount. I advise every client of mine to stay away from the hormone hoopla.

Herpes Havens

One of the worst traps of the beauty business is the newest trap of all. It's the current fad to ''try on'' sample cosmetics in department stores: Cosmetics which three thousand people before you have sampled . . . and heaven knows what two thousand of them were afflicted with. The newest disease of the generation, and the most irritating because it is incurable, is herpes—sores which are contagious. How in the world can you put products on your face, on your *mouth*, which have been touched before? Would you try on someone else's underwear?

If you are to have a makeup demonstration in a department store or in any public place make sure that the products used on your face are absolutely new and fresh—from an unopened container. Otherwise, say thanks-but-no-thanks to the ''free makeup.'' It could cost you for the rest of your life.

The pH Balance

There's a new game in town and that's the one that tells you you're doomed if your pH balance is disturbed. I wouldn't pay too much attention to the products that brag about their pH qualities: To me, it's just another example of media hype to sell you what you really don't need.

The pH balance is the acid–alkaline balance of the skin. Normal skin is slightly acidic with a pH somewhere between 5.5 and 6.8. Dissolved secretions of perspiration, oil, etc. cover the surface in what's known as an ''acid mantle.'' That's supposed to protect the skin. What's making many manufacturers wealthy is the theory that if you put anything on your face that's highly alkaline it can destroy the natural, protective balance. What the manufacturers don't tell you is that even if you do put a highly alkaline cleanser like detergent soap on your face the skin has a natural ability to bring itself back into balance soon after you remove the cleanser. The reason soap cleans so well is precisely because it has high alkaline properties, but it's not the alkaline that can hurt your skin so much as the perfumes and other chemicals in soaps. A product that advertises it protects the pH balance in your skin is giving away ice in the wintertime—something no one needs.

CHEAP IS CHEAP— THERE'S NO WAY AROUND IT

Margie buys her makeup at Woolworth's. ''It's exactly the same as the stuff you buy, Marilyn,'' she says, ''but your foundation comes in a silver box from Japan and it has a French name. So you pay three times as much.''

I've heard that song before and so have you. It's called Reverse Chic and it's a popular number. No wonder: Everyone loves to feel as if she's beaten the game. And sometimes the tune's not that far off key. Packaging costs and importing duties do add an enormous amount to cosmetics and when a certain line gains a good reputation you pay a whole lot extra for the name. No question. But somewhere in between there's a reasonable medium that has more truth than ''Cheap is exactly the same as big bucks.''

Buying cheap is a practice that sucks in as

many consumers as buying chicken placentas for pretty skin. First of all, the informed consumer has been had by beauty experts lately who have found it sells more books when they write that you can buy the same cosmetics at the five and dime, and what's more you can make them yourself from that old jello and cranberry juice that's been hanging out in your refrigerator for the last month. People feel absolutely brilliant and virtuous to discover a little-bucks substitute for the big-bucks expenditures. What's more, the irresistible buzz words that the industry is famous for—a mixture of scientific-sounding jargon and exotic frenchiness—are beginning to wear thin on a more informed public. Promises of ''cell awakening,'' ''millennium skin,'' ''les magiques eyes'' are sounding a little fishy—the industry's punishment for overkill. So, telling a woman she can find *cheap* les magiques is pretty good business, but it's not the truth—which, admittedly, is pretty hard to come by.

As someone who's spent half his career on the other side, the business side, of the beauty game, I can tell you that much of the truth; the important facts are withheld by the shakers and movers of the cosmetics industry. The industry tells you what it wants you to know about scientific research, about product information, and it's hard to make a really intelligent buying choice. Even though product labeling is supposed to tell you what you're buying, how many of us really know if glyceryl stearate, squalene or cetyl palmitate are useful or damaging? How do you know what long-term usage of a product will mean in terms of toxicity in the system? You really don't. You can be as much of a victim when talked into buying cheap products as you are when buying expensive.

Therefore, you have to use your common sense. And common sense tells you that, although of course there are exceptions, a company that spends more money on research dollars, on testing, will generally come up with better products than a company that, because it makes a smaller profit, simply cannot invest as much in trial and error. People expect you to deliver less when they pay less. On the whole, it has been my experience that, although you pay extra for status and glitter, it's true that the better products offer more. They don't cost a whole lot more—not ridiculous and unrealistic amounts more (suspect fraud when you come across irrational differences)—but as much as we'd like it to, quality generally never comes inexpensively.

I'll give you some examples. It's been my experience that cheap lipsticks dry out the lips. That's because their manufacturers put an inordinate amount of wax into the product. Companies which manufacture cheap products often claim that their budget prices come from paying less for salaries, promotion and training programs. I doubt that they do pay less for these expenditures: their top-level people, their enormous advertising programs cost plenty. The public is duped into thinking that because the salesperson at the five and dime makes less than the salesperson at the high-class department store, the extra money is poured back into the product. It's not.

Cheap mascaras may last long but try to get them off. What's more, because they are usually made from a synthetic plastic resin they make eyelashes look stiff and unnatural: It's like coating your lashes with plastic. Ever try a dollar-ninety-eight-cent gloss? Messy, greasy, sticky, non-lasting. One company puts out an all-purpose cocoa butter moisturizer that's supposed to be good for *all* skin types, oily through super-dry. Here's where your common sense should tell you something's wrong. No product can be all things to all people. So if it costs less than Revlon, it also does zilch for your skin if you happen to be over thirty and starting to dry out a bit. Moreover, it smells like cocoa butter—not wonderful for a face.

Check out the very-low-cost cosmetics in your five and dime. The colors, for the most part, are absolutely atrocious. That's because research is limited in these companies—all the profit goes to the manufacturer—and the color never went beyond Florentine Fuchsia which is cheap and easy to make. Subtlety, softness, attention to current color-fashion are virtually ignored. Can you really be happy with Screaming Orange even if it only costs two bucks? Can you find peace with Atavistic Aqua?

Low-priced cosmetics get away with a whole lot less quality than higher priced merchandise does. You feel funny complaining about the lack of moisture in a moisturizer that only set you back seventy-nine cents. I mean, "What do you expect for the price?" is the quite correct attitude. Woolworth's doesn't get many returns: You tend to make do with bargains. But, suddenly, your whole attitude changes when you've paid full dollar. If something doesn't measure up, you return it. Or else you should. So manufacturers, not loving that, tend to deliver at least half of what they promise, unlike the cheap manufacturers who can get away with a fourth of what they claim they can do.

I am convinced, despite the fact that I'm going against the tide by saying this, there are very few bargains in cosmetics. There are even fewer bargains in cosmetic tools. You can buy a cheap brush with which to apply powder or blusher, but learn to expect little

hairs over your lips and cheeks. You can try to apply your lipstick with an inexpensive lip brush, but be satisfied with hard, nonpliant brush hairs. Cosmetic brushes should be made of sable hair. Anything else doesn't last and performs poorly.

When you compute the cost of a cosmetic that lasts longer because of better ingredients than the dirt-cheap cosmetic, sometimes you end up saving money on the more expensive product. It happens all the time.

* Cheap foundations can irritate sensitive skin, come in a poor choice of colors, and don't blend easily.
* Cheap blushers don't last and can look waxy.
* Cheap mascaras run, irritate the eyes, are stiff and tend to clump and dry out.
* Cheap powders often have color added, give pasty, ricecake textures.
* Cheap eye shadows irritate, congeal in creases, cake up, don't blend and come in garish colors.
* Cheap lipsticks are either mushy soft or waxy hard, don't have staying power and often taste like poison.
* Cheap creams, including moisturizers and eye creams, are full of oils, perfumes and alcohols.

It's usually a no-win situation, the bargain cosmetic. On the other hand, sometimes you find a line that's not cheap, not expensive, just reasonable. The packaging is modest in these lines, depend on it, and the origin is usually local. Rest assured that you will not find abrasive soap in the cleansing lotions of these lines, or heavy perfumes in the foundations. That's because the manufacturer has respect for her clients. Estée Lauder and Clinique are, in my opinion, two such companies on whose products one can usually rely.

If you have found the miracle El Cheapo I'd like to know about it.

*

So much for the bad news: The truth will make you free, as they say. Now for the good news. Once you've learned how to bypass the hyped-up cosmetic and skin-care products your next job is to learn how to bring into being the meticulously clean, relatively lump-, bump- and fleck-free canvas on which to paint your makeup colors. You have to. Your makeup is only as good as the skin to which you apply it. It would be nice if you could conceal poor skin with makeup over-doses, but take it from me, you can't. It's essential, therefore, to clean up your skin act and learn how to maintain that clean canvas.

2 *

Saving Face: Skin Care and Maintenance

BEFORE EMBARKING on any new skin care program you ought to have a clear idea of your goals and the obstacles to those goals. If your goal is to make beautiful skin that will do justice to beautiful makeup you ought to think of that skin as a machine—a system of many working parts that thrives when the system is well lubricated and free of dirt and breaks down when the parts are clotted with debris. In order to have a clean machine it won't do to service it with a slap of soap, a splash of water. You ought to get *under* the surface to root out debris because surface purity relies on under-the-surface purity. What is under there that needs so much servicing? None other than:

BLACKHEADS, WHITEHEADS AND ZITS

Sounds like a law firm, I know, but blackheads, whiteheads and zits don't do any good for anybody (as opposed to lawyers, who do). They're the end results of a substance known as sebum, a viscous liquid composed of pus and oil that begins to be produced in the sebaceous glands at puberty. While increased hormone production at puberty does splendid things for burgeoning sexuality it doesn't do a whole lot for the complexion. Sebaceous glands get a booster shot from puberty and they react by really turning on the juice (or oil, in this case). The oil is normally released through skin pores but sometimes, with all that action, the pores get blocked. A blackhead is a little round mass, a plug that collects when the pore is blocked. Eventually it nudges open the pore and when the cells at the plug's surface hit the air they oxidize, solidify and turn black. Blackheads, thus, do not come from dirt, no matter what your mother told you. Everyone, even Princess Di, has blackheads, and you know how clean and refined her pores must be.

Sometimes it happens that the same pores are tightly closed and the sebum doesn't hit the air, oxidize and turn black. Instead it stays captured under the skin. In this case, you have a whitehead (sometimes called a closed comedo), not that much more terrific than a blackhead. And sometimes, bacteria or even friction from squeezing and other abrasive acts breaks up the sebum into many small units which explode follicle walls, spread to adjoining pores and turn into various types of skin lesions. These lesions are known to the medical and beauty experts as pustules, nodules and cysts (no, not another law firm) and to adolescents the world over as zits. Zits are really the pits. They do *not* come from chocolate, nuts, dirt or bad thoughts. They come primarily from growing up—the same as blackheads and whiteheads—when pores are blocked by excess oil production.

In order to avoid blocked pores, you have to surface-clean your skin gently and systematically and then maintain that cleanliness with a deep-cleaning regimen that does not rely on machines or skin-irritating treatments. And that's why this section of the book is crucial. Makeup is irrelevant if your skin's not a clean machine. Here, then, is the Skin-Care Two-Step—the STS.

THE SKIN-CARE TWO-STEP

I feel as if I should start with a trumpet call, what I have to tell you here is so important. It's taken years of research, observation and practice but I've finally got it! I know how to make your skin look fantastic.

Throw out all the beauty books that promise baby skin with baby-talk that gurgles on about acupuncture, vaporizing, ultraviolet lights, good thoughts and visits to the Great Skin Doctor God. The truth is that the only way you can reconstitute dull, pimpled or prematurely aging skin is by cleanliness—on the surface and under the surface. I've devised a system that takes care of both. That's the good news.

Now for the bad news. You've paid a lot of money for this book and you're entitled to results and truth. You *will* get results from using my system, but the results are not of the instant variety. Your skin cannot metamorphose from bad or mediocre skin to great skin overnight. As a matter of fact—here's the killer—your skin will definitely get worse before it gets better. It has to. There's no way to get great skin instantly. You can't peel off blackheads and pimples as you can lift specks of dust off velvet with a little Scotch tape—no matter how many lies to the contrary you've been buying up till now. It takes construction and a little time to push those impurities to the surface and out of the skin, and in the process your face will *show* it's working hard. There's no way around it. But it's crazy to throw away money on wonderful paints until you've cleaned the canvas. The enchantment of makeup is richest, most appealing, on nice skin.

But then, here's more good news. Once you get rid of the splotches and blotches and have suffered through a day or so (it's not so terrible, really) of working skin, your face should be reborn. It will look splendid. It will look dewier. If you have lines, they will be muted. If you had areas of blemishes, they will be gone (or almost gone). Your skin will be prepared for you to play with the wonder of makeup.

You can't clean the canvas with soap, no matter how pretty the Ivory Girl looks. Soap can decrease natural facial oil by as much as one third, drying your skin to a sand-like texture. And don't rely on the "special soaps" either. Soap and useless panaceas are out. Forget the steaming, scrubbing, estrogen, antibiotics, health foods, broccoli creams, liquid-soap dispensers and other hyped-up offerings of the charlatans which promise you instant magic. You can even throw your new fire and ice treatment out the window. It will probably only burn and freeze your skin.

What *will* do it? The Skin-Care Two-Step—a two-step affair to clean and wonderful skin.

Step 1: The Night Moves
Step 2: The Maintenance Moves

If you follow the Step 1 process before sleep each night (it will only take five minutes) and supplement it with Step 2 each week (it will only take about an hour, total), your skin *must* improve. It's the simplest, most logical plan in the world. Do the Two-Step. I stake my entire career upon your good results.

Step 1: The Night Moves

Make them every night; they consist of

* Cleanser
* Freshener
* Moisturizer
* Eye Cream

CLEANSER

You must take off your makeup and the day's grime before you go to sleep. If you do nothing else to preserve your skin, this is an absolute necessity. Even if you go to bed with the most fabled lover in the world and you want to look terrific *in* your makeup, you'd better wake up an hour after the festivities to get that makeup off. It's that important.

The same kind of cleanser should work for *everyone.* You will be inundated with advertisements about milky lotions versus granular lotions versus fruit lotions. Ignore them

all. A cleansing cream or lotion should not be heavy with soap (which is the very thing you're trying to avoid by using the cleanser). A cleansing lotion should not be an irritant. It should not contain alcohol or grains to aggravate sensitive skin. I use a whipped aloe and collagen cleanser for everyone. It doesn't dry, it doesn't abrade, it doesn't make you smell like a brothel, it doesn't make you taste like an avocado, it doesn't promise you everlasting happiness. It cleans. Thoroughly.

If you wear contact lenses, remove them. Apply the cleanser all over your face and to your eyes. Leave the cleanser on while you brush your teeth or tweeze the stray hair from your brow. This gives it a chance to emulsify, break down the makeup and raise the dirt from the pores. Instead of tissuing away endlessly, waiting a minute or so for the cleanser to do its work allows you to remove the cleanser, sebum and makeup effortlessly with a tissue. Follow up with a warm washcloth.

There's a myth going the rounds that says because tissues are a product derived from wood, tiny wood grains can be left on your face to enter the pores as you wipe your face clean. Absolute nonsense, and yet another example of media hysteria. It's the same mentality that says you should apply and remove your makeup in upward strokes to prevent skin sagging. If you follow that advice, you'll be removing makeup until next Halloween. When you sleep and press your head in the pillow, it's hardly in an upward-strokes-only position. Taking off makeup—in any direction—will not do more or less to prevent wrinkles or skin sag.

Here are some cleansers that I've found to be consistently effective. If you don't already have your own favorites, you might give them a try.

✻ Chanel Démaquillant Doux Cleanser
✻ Lancôme Galatée Milky Creme Cleanser

There are special and effective ways to remove mascara. If mascara is *not* waterproof, water or a nonoily liquid eye-makeup remover will do the trick. If it is waterproof, you need an oily or creamy textured remover. Plain cold cream should also do the job. Vaseline or thick oil like Johnson's Baby Oil may make a bigger mess than the whole thing warrants. I usually use this procedure:

Enclose your index finger in a tissue and place it under your lower lashes, then dip a Q-Tip into the removing material, close your eyes and wipe both sets of lashes. The Q-Tip removes most of the upper-lash color and the lower-lash color comes off on the tissue, not in your eye. Repeat with a clean Q-Tip until the lashes are clean. Also clean under the lashes with a Q-Tip.

FRESHENER

Pat on some freshener with a cotton ball and allow it to dry. This tones and removes any traces of dirt left by the cleanser. If the freshener has no alcohol in it, you can use it around the eyes as well. I do advise, for all skin types, a freshener without alcohol; it adds nothing except excess drying. However, Clinique puts out an effective freshener containing alcohol (marketed as "cosmetic alcohol," implying it's milder) and acetone (a solvent), which should be used only on very oily, nonsensitive skin, even though it's labeled for "normal to partly oily skin." By the way, depending on the manufacturer's whim, freshener can be called astringent, toner or clarifying lotion.

Here are two fresheners you might decide to try.

✻ Clinique Clarifying Lotion 2 (oily, nonsensitive skin)
✻ Elizabeth Arden Moisture Action

MOISTURIZER

You do need a lubricating cream before you go to sleep so it can work its magic all night. The cream I prefer consists of aloe and collagen which will be beautifully absorbed as it nourishes and softens the skin's frown and smile lines. Think of it as a skin meal or a skin drink. Even if you have oily skin don't cringe at the idea of a moisturizing night cream. The best moisturizers contain no or very little oil which cannot be absorbed easily or which just sits there clogging surface pores. Moisturizers should contain water to hydrate (provide moisture)—quite a different animal from oil. It's best applied when the skin is damp so it can seal in that moisture.

Many manufacturers put out special heavy night creams: You don't need a *heavy* moisturizer. You need a product that can be used day or night (I often call it a dermal-feeder) and which will mellow existing lines and act as a retardant against the formation of others. No cream will take away wrinkles. Check the list of ingredients on moisturizer products you are considering: If oil is listed near the top you know the product is heavy with the greasy stuff. Here are some moisturizers I've found effective in the past.

✻ Clinique Dramatically Different Moisturizing Lotion
✻ Clinique Very Emollient Cream (very concentrated, for very dry skins—use only a drop or so)
✻ Doak Pharmacal Formula 405 Light Textured Moisturizer
✻ Estée Lauder Re-Nutriv

SAVING FACE: SKIN CARE AND MAINTENANCE

* Progrès Plus Creme Anti-Rides
* Revlon Eterna '27' (use only a drop or so)

EYE CREAM

There are three portions of the body that contain very few oil ducts: the palms of the hands, the soles of the feet and the eye area. As a result, they wrinkle quite easily and in the case of the eyes, which are involved in every normal facial expression, this could spell premature aging of the whole face. What's the solution? Again, a moisturizing cream, but this time, one specially formulated for the paper-thin tissue that surrounds the eye. Regular face cream has a thicker, more concentrated consistency than eye cream and tends to blow up the area around the eye when applied there. So I suggest the lighter, more easily absorbed eye cream.

Apply the cream around the eyes, owl fashion, and out to the temples. It should look like the Lone Ranger's mask except it won't go over the bridge of the nose. Caution: Don't spoon out dollops of the stuff: A little goes a long way. Below are three eye creams I recommend.

* Clarins (Boume, not Gel)
* Elizabeth Arden Bye-Lines
* Ultima CHR

That's it! Clean your face, apply a freshener, a moisturizer and finally, an eye cream. Those are the Night Moves of the Skin-Care Two-Step, the simplest and most effective cleansing and moisturizing treatment in the world. It's taken five minutes, three of which were spent brushing your teeth—which you'd be doing anyway, please God.

This is the major part of the cleansing routine. You will need only these short steps to insure wonderful skin on the four or five days a week that you don't have to worry about the maintenance moves (which follow). When you wake up every morning, you will only need the most minimal of cleansing care before you apply makeup.

Go to bed. Tomorrow you'll deal with Step 2 of the STS.

Step 2: The Maintenance Moves

Make them two or three times a week; they consist of

* Exfoliation
* Ejection

After you learn how to cleanse and moisturize (Step 1), you have to supplement with a maintenance plan. That means facials. I know how difficult it is to find time for facials after a busy day, but no one is lazier than I, and if I can find a half hour two or three times a week to care for my own oil-troubled skin, so can you. Used in conjunction with Step 1, a facial will ventilate, expurgate and give new, surging health to your skin. *It has to work*. Facials, unlike the daily cleaning and moisturizing process, go deeper.

EXFOLIATION

This is the removal, by cream and light massage, of the dead cells that sit on the surface of the skin. Let me explain: According to the dictionary, exfoliate means "to throw off scales and flakes." The skin is composed of several different layers and the layer that is visible to anyone looking at you, the outermost layer, is called the epidermis. Incredibly enough, it replaces itself every month with the used cells flaking off—a kind of dandruff, if you will. All of these used cells don't fall conveniently and invisibly to the floor, though. They tend to just sit there on the skin blocking a naturally healthy glow. These dead flakes of skin also have another wonderful trick: They tend to embed themselves in facial lines, making the lines seem more like sidewalk cracks than slight indentations. The last, and probably the worst thing that flakes left too long on the skin can do is act like manhole covers on the pores, shutting in the blackheads and other impurities that need to escape. Those manhole covers must be raised. The skin, after all, is an organ of elimination and pores should be kept open. That's why makeup companies which sell facial masques without exfoliants are doing a huge disservice to their clients. The masque without the exfoliant is just another manhole cover. Men who shave are in essence exfoliating their skin. "They are giving themselves a minidermabrasion," says Dr. Nia K. Terezakis, assistant professor of clinical dermatology at Tulane Medical School, "and those men have better skin than those who do not shave every day." Precisely my point.

Exfoliators can be called scrubs, grains, buffers, abrasive sponges or peeling creams. The latter is the best and most gentle. I use an aloe-based cream to avoid any possible allergic reactions, but you can experiment with different, gentle creams from other lines such as Lancôme's Bienfait Démaquillant. I caution you *never* to use a mechanical exfoliator or even any abrasive "applicator" products like the popular Buf-Puf which, in my opinion, can be damaging if used too enthusiastically. Products like these tend to buff your skin to glowing rawness, happily breaking capillaries along the way. What's a

broken capillary? You'll know one when you meet one. They're those red, spider-like lines around the nose especially; minute blood vessels that have been broken by pressure. Wine often tends to expand and dilate capillaries also, which is why you'll see those tiny red lines around the nose of a heavy drinker.

What follows next is the process you must use to exfoliate—to throw off the scales and flakes of the outer layer of skin. First, a good skin-peeling cream must be applied to a freshly cleansed face.

1. Carefully *pat* the cream on, all over the face up to the temples and hair line, carefully avoiding the eyes.

2. Keep yourself busy for ten minutes while the cream sets.

3. Dampen your fingertips after the ten minutes and gently massage the exfoliant (it will have gained the consistency of toothpaste) off the face. As the cream comes off, so will the dead skin flakes.

4. Pat clean with a washcloth and warm water to remove all traces of exfoliant from the skin.

EJECTION

After getting rid of the outer layer of dead skin, you must get the bad stuff that's *under* the skin up and out. That's where the masque comes in. The idea behind the masque is to constrict the pores. It surrounds, pushes up and gets out the impurities. My favorite is a camomile, aloe and collagen masque, which my own chemist makes up. You can also purchase aloe and collagen products in many department stores and cosmetic specialty shops because the ingredients appear in many of the better cosmetics lines. Camomile is a fragrant herb that has been used for centuries for its curative qualities. Aloe is the juice of the succulent plant called an *aloe vera*. It never dies because it produces its own life-giving gel called aloe vera gel, which heals and nourishes (it contains amino acids and carbohydrates) and also appears to aid the collagen ingredient in my masque to penetrate deeply into the skin. This is important because collagen, a protein substance found in the body's connective tissues, allays wrinkling and aging of the skin.

Now I have heard—I must be honest—hundreds of grim-faced dermatologists proclaim that collagen and aloe cannot penetrate past the outer layer of skin. I totally reject that theory. Science changes its mind every twenty minutes and so do holders of medical degrees, which is why I don't pay too much attention to the latter in matters of skin care. While the nay-sayers are saying nay, the collagen goes on sinking deeply into the skin, creating silken softness every step of the way. The aloe also penetrates and helps promote the growth of healthy skin cells just as it stimulates the growth of tissue to help heal wounds. Dermatologists say aloe is comprised mostly of water. Tell that to the thousands of burn victims who have been gratefully healed by the wonderful succulent. Tell that to the hundreds of my clients who swear by its nonhormonal cell-rejuvenating qualities. It *is* absorbed and it *does* work. I think the use of aloe and collagen is like watering a plant: You have to nourish the roots to keep the leaves healthy.

You may choose your own masque—it doesn't have to be my camomile, aloe and collagen combination. Whatever you choose, the masque must condition the skin, constrict the pores and guide the sebum-filled blemishes to the surface. Experiment with different products to find one you like, but stay away from the heavily astringent and oil-based products which may flay the skin and clog the pores. Here are two products you might try.

* Chattem Laboratories Mudd Super Cleansing Treatment
* Shiseido (the rinse-off masque, not the peel-off one)

To apply a masque for the purpose of ejection:

1. Pat the cream all over your freshly cleansed and exfoliated face and put a little on the neck area also.

2. Take your phone off the hook. This is not just piquant advice. While you won't develop a severe case of lockjaw, as the masque tightens your mouth won't work quite normally, possibly alarming your mother. While

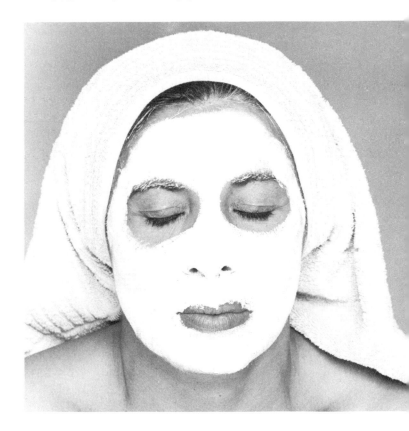

you're relaxing for the sybaritic ten minutes the masque is not just sitting there on top of your skin. It's being absorbed; it's tightening and constricting the pores; it's surrounding, getting under and pushing the impurity out. In short, it's doing its job. Anything in those pores that doesn't belong there is slowly being pushed toward the surface. Because the masque is cool, it constricts rapidly.

3. After ten minutes wet a washcloth with warm water (never an extreme of hot or cold which is murder on capillaries), wash the masque off, apply freshener and moisturizer to your face and neck, and an eye cream.

4. Go to sleep.

That's it. You should feel positively virtuous because you've done a splendid thing for yourself. It's a good idea to enjoy your facial before you go to bed so the skin has a chance to breathe deeply, without makeup, all night long.

The whole thing has taken less than half an hour. The visible results (remember I mentioned bad news?) will soon be, somewhat unpleasantly, apparent.

IN THE MORNING   Okay, here it is—the unpleasant part. You'll notice two distinct changes in your face this morning.

First, check out those dry areas of the face where the lines and crevices have always been heaviest: They should look quite a bit smoother because the exfoliant has removed the layer of dead skin that has been sitting in those lines, deepening them. Not only does exfoliation seem to smooth out wrinkles, but the suctioning action of the masque also results in less firmly embedded lines. Light can now reflect on the face where it couldn't yesterday. There seems to be a moister, fresher look. Please understand, the facial cannot re-move lines, but it can mute them, making them far less obvious.

The second change is not going to make me popular with you. Your face has not looked quite so *active* in ages. Any blackheads you've had under the surface are now peeking out; any sebaceous cysts (those tiny little bumps under the skin) will now have minuscule whiteheads on them; redness will be the most prevalent color. Everything, as they say, is now up front. Okay, despair a little, but then rejoice! Just what you wanted to happen is happening. You're getting all that junk out, out, out of your face. Don't worry about how it looks. Just use a little foundation and powder to cover up the battlefield as well as you can and don't schedule the audition for today. *Whatever you do*—no matter how tempted you are—*don't squeeze!* I don't care if you hang ribbons on, bronze or take pictures of those raised and reddened pimples—just don't squeeze!

Pinching and digging at your face creates scars and infections. Your face, though a little ravaged, is not an archaeological site to be excavated. Your facial is working if your skin looks annoyed. You can't keep suppressing pus and excess oil under the skin and expect it to evanesce magically into the air. Sometimes dermatologists prescribe an assortment of medication to "clear up" the skin. In my experience what that most often accomplishes is to keep the sebum under the skin, which controls the disorder for a while, but which *doesn't cure*. It doesn't get to the root of the problem. If you have been meticulous about skin care and maintenance, and a problem still exists, *then* try a drying lotion for your breakouts. May I make this suggestion? Only spot the lotion on where it is necessary. Do not apply it broadly over skin that is relatively clear.

BLACKHEAD EMERGENCY FIXES

Five to Try

* Regular cleansing and facial treatments prevent blackheads but sometimes a stray one appears just around the nose where pores become particularly dilated from the larger oil glands. Wet a washcloth with warm water and apply it to the area to loosen the blackhead plug. Do this for about five minutes. Then, with fingertips wrapped in tissue, gently *press* (don't squeeze hard) the plug out. Do this only for emergencies; regular pressure can widen the pores permanently and break capillaries, and squeezing and picking can permanently scar skin. Avoid like the plague the "special comedone extractors." They're the *worst*.

* Never steam your face in a container that sends hot steam directly to it. If blackheads appear, you can try steaming them out in a steam *room* or even in a long, hot shower. That softens the plugs and enables you to gently press them out. If they won't come out with pressing, don't squeeze. You know the difference. Take an extra exfoliating and facial treatment. Don't try a steam room for pimples, cysts or whiteheads—it won't work. The pore openings in these blemishes are too small for the sebum to escape.

* If your skin is not very dry, try an over-the-counter pad medicated with salicylic acid (like Stri-Dex Medicated Pads): blackheads and whiteheads sometimes respond to the substance.

* Try an over-the-counter benzyl peroxide (only a 5 percent solution should be used for small pimples and blackheads; a 10 percent dosage is too strong for faces), apply a dab to the blackhead for about two or three hours, every night for a week. After the three hours, rinse the benzyl peroxide off. Remember: Don't put the peroxide all over your face, only *spot*-treat it.

* Add an extra exfoliation treatment to your regular skin-care program. Exfoliation not only peels off dead cuticle, it opens up follicular channels so the oil and sebum can drain out (along with the blackheads).

Two to Avoid

* If your dermatologist suggests a round of X-ray therapy for an acne condition or a blackhead breakout, say, "Thanks, but no thanks." It's drastic and potentially very harmful treatment.

* Be very wary about ultraviolet treatments. Many skin doctors now say they cause more harm than good. But plain old sun? Why not?

What Happens Next?

In two or three days, you'll give yourself another facial. As you exfoliate your pores will widen. The blackheads will begin to come out on your fingertips, looking like sprinkled pepper. The whiteheads that were on the sebaceous cyst will be naturally abraded by the exfoliant; little drops of liquid inside the cysts will come out and the little bubbles of skin will begin to recede back to the natural skin line. Your face will not look wonderful yet, but after this second facial you'll soon begin to see a marked improvement in your complexion. The two-day blotched skin hiatus will be memory and well worth the smoother future of your face. So, think of the line, "My skin *must* get worse before it gets better"—think of the end results.

In the next few days, your skin should appear more limpid, sunnier, younger than ever before. Don't get overly confident. Skin care requires tenacity. You have to keep after your complexion for the rest of your life. It's really not such a big price to pay. When you consider the two facials weekly that dry skin needs (about forty-five minutes total) and the three facials weekly that oily skin needs (a little more than an hour), then there is no one, not the biggest executive, debutante or homemaker, who should deny herself facial clarity for the cost, in time, of that hour or so a week.

A regular skin cleansing program must be combined with a regular exfoliation and facial program. The latter does for your face what the newly popular Nautilus equipment does for the body—tones it and allows it to develop to its fullest potential.

You can buy pounds of the most extraordinary cosmetics and you can buy hours with expensive makeup artists, and your makeup will still be only as good as the skin to which you apply it. Cleansing, moisturizing and deep-cleaning facials go together. Once you get into the Skin-Care Two-Step you will take a hedonistic, sensuous pleasure in caring for your skin. On top of all else, it is a nurturing, relaxing experience.

My program is a winner. It really is. Not magic, not wishful thinking—the STS will work, if you work at it.

∗

In order to know how many facials a week you'll need, you must know what kind of skin you have. But, despite the compact, cut-and-dried charts you see in most makeup books, analysis of your skin is not quite so cut-and-dried.

THE SKIN YOU'RE IN

The skin you're in—is it dry? Oily? Simply terrific? Don't be so sure. Skin's fickle. It changes with the seasons, with your age, even with day-to-day differences. The oily skin you have today may shock you tomorrow after a day at the ski resort by drying up and acting more fragile than you ever dreamed possible. That's really okay, you know. In fact, in a way it's really quite wonderful. Your skin, like your personality or your dreams, should never remain static.

What's Your Skin Type?

Below is a guide—not an irrevocable analysis—so you should treat it as one. Anyone who labels her skin from a book with the certainty that the label is as steadfast as her eye color is in for a shock. The best you can do is to get an idea of your skin type today, or at best, for this season of your life.

AN OILY SKIN?

* Do you have enlarged pores?
* Do you seem to need daily shampoos because your hair is so oily?
* Are your pores enlarged when you check in a magnifying mirror?
* Do you have a tendency to acne or blackheads?
* Do you tan easily?
* Are you olive or sallow in complexion?
* If you looked at your nose right now, would it be shining?
* Do you find that you have to clean your face *meticulously:* one slip-up means a breakout?

Are most of your answers yes? Then your skin, these days, is an oily skin.

A DRY SKIN?

* When you look in a magnifying mirror are your pores almost invisible?
* Can you get away with a hair wash every two or three days?
* Does your skin tend to itch, flake, get chapped?
* Do you get sunburn very easily?
* Do you have tiny splits in your facial skin that hurt?
* Do you have very tiny, premature wrinkle lines around your mouth or eyes?
* Do you often have broken capillaries or spidery red lines showing through?
* Is your skin kind of transparent?
* Do you rarely have zits?
* Do you have freckles?
* Does your skin stay red for more than a second after you pinch it?
* If you pinch your neck skin out, does it kind of wait a second or so before jumping back on your neck?
* Is your skin dry to the touch, with a very flat texture?

Are most of your answers yes? Then your skin, these days, is a dry skin.

A NORMAL SKIN?

* Do you hardly ever have dandruff?
* Is your skin supple, flexible, smooth in texture?
* Does your makeup stay on without congealing or getting blotchy or oily?
* Do you tan slowly?
* Would you say that you hardly ever get pimples except, perhaps, around the time of your menstrual period or when you know you haven't cleaned your face properly?
* Is your complexion neither extremely fair nor extremely dark toned, but somewhere in the middle?

Are most of your answers yes? Then your skin, these days is a normal or even a combination skin: It's almost always fairly good.

Checkpoint!

You've determined the skin you're in—today. What kinds of changes in diet, environment, exercise and aging can be the checkpoints that determine your skin's status—tomorrow? Consider the chart below and see how to best care for your skin today so it will be simply terrific tomorrow. It's your move: Checkmate! The checkpoint chart is the smartest strategy in town for the woman who really knows how to play the skin game.

Skin Savers

Consider them life savers for your skin. You can pluck them from your own environment. They make your whole body, as well as your face, feel new, and they're free and easy. I offer you five tried-and-true skin savers. If you practice at least three daily, you'll notice a definite difference in skin tone and texture.

CHECKPOINT CHANGE	WHAT CAN IT DO?	**WHAT SHOULD YOU DO?** If you have oily skin
SUN OVERDOSES *(Never, never use a sun reflector for a tan—no matter what kind of skin you have.)*	Bring wrinkles, dry skin; burned skin; can cause changes in pigmentation; can cause skin cancer.	Intelligent sun doses can't hurt—may even dry up your pimples; use sun block but you can get away with low SPF (sun protection factor). Moisturize after sun exposure.
PREGNANCY *(Blotches, darkened scars often disappear after giving birth; moles can be surgically removed after giving birth.)*	Early in pregnancy: speeds up oil production. Late in pregnancy: possible moles, blotches, blood vessel breakage, pigmentation darkening (chloasma), hair loss.	Intensify cleaning and facial regimen. Drink water in large amounts; avoid caffeine.
STEAM HEAT	Dry skin about as much as the Sahara Desert would: A lot!	Moisturize more often; drink more water.
WIND, COLD, ICE	Toughen the horny outer layer of skin; dry skin; can burn and chap.	Avoid extremes of cold or hot water; moisturize more often; be sure you use lip protector; protect exposed face with long scarf or mask if wind is really severe; rinse soap from skin *completely*.
PASSING YEARS	Oil production slows up and skin becomes dryer; tiny lines and wrinkles appear; skin becomes more sensitive, more fragile.	Clean more often. If you've always used soap, this may be the time you have to begin using cleansing lotion instead to forestall drying. Your skin will definitely weather better than dryer skin, but moisturize anyway.
DIETS	Unbalanced diets can dry your skin from water loss, can cause pallor, or fragile skin. Yo-yo dieting (lose some, gain some in steady patterns) can stretch your skin and cause it to sag. Diuretics that drain water from your skin may cause it to wrinkle prematurely. Vitamin C deficiencies can cause easy bruising; Vitamin E deficiencies can create delayed healing of hurt skin; Vitamins B complex, C and E deficiencies can contribute to hair loss. (Remember—eating chocolate, fried foods, oily or greasy foods may not be fabulous for your body, but they don't give you acne.)	*Never* deal with all or nothing fad diets: they're poor for every kind of skin. Too much water can puff your skin out, too little can wrinkle it. Prolonged fasting is anathema to all skin. Diets should be varied and vitamin supplements should be taken (on advice from physician or nutritionist) to replace lost nourishment.
AIR POLLUTION	Spending long periods of time in "dirty" environments can cause skin infections from combination of oil and dirt; chemicals in dirty air can dry and age.	Must cleanse more often. A *very* mild soap is okay to use. If pollution is very bad, try a light astringent toner to remove oily dirt, after regular cleansing.

If you have dry skin

Take in *very* small doses; use sun block with very high (10–15) sun protective factor (SPF); use light foundation base when out in sun—even when just walking around. Moisturize before, during and after sun exposure. Wear protective clothing.

Stay out of sun as much as possible; moisturize more often; avoid perfumes or cosmetics with perfumes; avoid strong soaps (any soaps, actually).

Keep pan of water near heat source; sleep with vaporizer or humidifier; pile on the moisturizer; spray face with water-atomizer.

Use a deep-penetrating moisturizer; after skiing, sledding, add *extra* cream. Stay far away from the après-ski fire; intense heat following wind and cold can definitely break blood vessels. Avoid drying soaps; apply moisture during the day to under-eye, around mouth area. Ski masks that cover the whole face are great when planning long winter exposure; stay away from all exposure; stay away from all astringents (especially any with alcohol). On mouth, apply baby oil, Vaseline, any really protective cream before going skiing, skating, etc. Use a sun block cream when glare is present.

Clean meticulously to rid skin of drying and dead skin cells; moisturize *very* often; never go out without a moisturizer or foundation to protect skin from elements; exfoliate more often and use lubricating face masques each time.

Must cleanse more often but all that washing can dehydrate skin; use mild cleansing lotions and nonoily light moisturizers; be careful to avoid more chemicals or astringents that will strip the skin of whatever oil it has.

If you have normal—combo skin

Build up exposure from fifteen minutes to maximum exposure; use moisturizer before and after and a sun block with medium (5-9) SPF. Wear a hat to protect your face.

Sleep, eat well, use sun block with high SPF; clear nail polish keeps nails strong; use hair conditioner to combat dry hair.

Drink water, moisturize at least twice daily; use humidifier during the day; try to turn off heat in P.M.

Spot moisturizer on regularly during the day where you need it most. Extra conditioner on hair is useful. At night, make sure skin is damp before applying moisturizer; avoid long tub soaks (they dry, especially if the water is hot).

Never use products with alcohol or heavy perfume; moisturize more often; avoid extremes of sun and wintry blasts.

Use special gentle eye cream (after cleansing) more often to avoid drying of this area. Collagen creams are useful to dry and combo-skin to combat drying from extra cleansing.

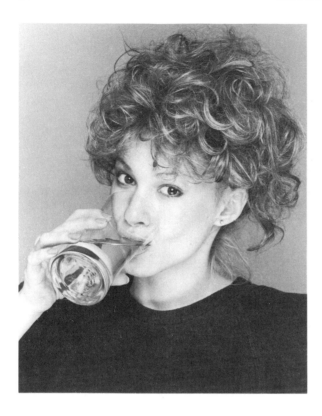

THE WATER FACTOR

Plain water, used inside and out, is a better present for your skin than emeralds. Because it's free, very few women buy it or trust its usefulness. Those in the know quietly go about creating cherubic skin for themselves with water. Take Christie Brinkley, who confides, "Water is my secret weapon; I put it in the air I breathe, I drink it and I apply it to my skin. At night I sleep with a vaporizer. And I spray mineral water on my face before using a moisturizer." Another million-dollar model, Cristina Ferrare, says, "I drink eight glasses of room temperature water each day to get rid of skin impurities."

Drinking water is a purge. It purifies the bloodstream by cleansing it of all contaminations. It helps your kidneys to flush out burned fats and other wastes. It's even a good idea to drink a glass of water before meals (despite what your mother told you) because the temporary feeling of fullness you get can be a great diet aid. Water retention does not come from drinking water: on the contrary, drinking water rids your body of fluids. Eating salty products is what causes the tissues to retain water. The purified blood flows to your face and gives your skin a glow and health you cannot duplicate! You're allowed to alternate plain water with iced tea, club soda and other variations. Since you lose about two quarts of water a day (about a quart through urination, one to three pints through sweating, another pint just from breathing) you should drink about six to eight glasses every day.

Make a facial water-spray by putting mineral water into a sterilized glass spray-bottle and treat yourself to a nourishing water spritz *at least* in the morning and before you put on your evening moisturizing cream. Christie's idea of using a vaporizer (a cold water vaporizer, not the stifling, steam heat variety) while she sleeps is excellent. It's all-night, no-work skin moisturizing.

A tip: Occasionally, when water-flushing your system, and especially as you get older, you may notice a "puffy-morning-face" syndrome. As the body lies flat in bed, fluid sometimes drains into the face. To solve this raise the head of your bed four inches by propping books underneath the bed's wheels or boxspring. It's also a healthier way to sleep.

A word of caution: Drinking water is not the same as sitting in it. Even though many spas extol long hot-tub baths, hours of soaking in particularly hot water dissolves the skin's own lipids which protect it from the drying effects of the environment. What's too long to stay in the bath? Is your skin drying, swelling or cracking? Is it puckering over your fingernails? Are you lobster-red? Are you bored witless? It's too long. Drink. Spray. Don't soak.

THE SEXUAL FACTOR

Don't laugh and don't knock it. Sex is good for a whole lot of things and it's particularly good for your skin. The orgasmic flush sends all that blood racing toward your face, spurring on circulation, lowering the blood cholesterol level and making you look radiant and renewed. Your complexion thrives on the sexual flush and as many as you can manage without seeming greedy is like skin manna. Good sex combines the skin-saving benefits of aerobic exercise (without its bone jarring effects) with its unique stress-relieving benefits. Try sex. You'll like it.

THE EXERCISE FACTOR

Your well-being, your physical suppleness will not only unkink the muscles, help your heart and jog your breathing, it will also—you better believe it—bring that healthy, reborn look to your skin. First of all, when you exercise you're perspiring—which enlarges those pores and helps the impurities in the skin to escape. Second, exercise fuels the body with revved-up circulation: It livens up every muscle, every cell—especially the facial ones. It's always been very clear to me that there are definite connections between facial clarity and body health and deep breathing. Stingy movers and breathers have sluggish, congestive, even toxic systems and it shows on the face every time. A fine kind of exercise is aerobic exercise—movement that makes use of oxygen, of deep breathing. Any skin care product that tells you to sit in front of a mirror and make funny little grimaces to exercise the facial muscles is not worth the money you're paying for it. Only improved blood circulation truly exercises facial and other muscles in a meaningful way. So, pick an activity and build up to, at the very least, a three-times-a-week workout. We're talking a half an hour now, three times or more a week. We're talking tennis, swimming, jogging, aerobic dancing, ballet dancing or even brisk walking. We're talking *moving*. The skin reflects the body's general fitness and health. I can tell by looking at the skin color, tone and texture of a client if she's had enough sleep, exercise, even happiness. And of the three, I believe that exercise counts most for glowing skin. It's the best base in the world for makeup.

A tip: if your circulation is really sluggish, it may show up in dark circles under your eyes where fragile skin shows it first.

THE RELAXATION FACTOR

You may not know it, but there's no way to stop tenseness from being mirrored on your face. Had a bad day? Your mouth imperceptibly tightens, pulling the skin, creating tiny little lines around the corners of your mouth and eyes. They're not laugh lines, either. Someone didn't pay you? Your lips are tightly closed as you go about your business, drawing that skin, artificially aging it. When there are periods of emotional stress or even deep concentration, your skin may be the loser. It broadcasts information that's actually no one else's business—what kind of a night it was, what kind of a business deal you made.

Skin conditions like psoriasis, eczema and acne can be worsened by stress. Your skin can actually produce more oil in times of tension because the adrenal glands become overactive, the hormone balance changes and voilà!—oily facial secretions and pimples. Stress can also set the stage for infection and allergy, leading causes of skin disorders. Take a fifteen-minute chunk from every day and hone your relaxation skills during it.

Relaxation techniques may include massage, head rolls, personal mantras, yoga, transcendental meditation. The best thing you can do is go to a library and research some of the easily learned self-relaxation techniques.

THE VITAMIN FACTOR

Beware the taking of vitamins indiscriminately. Many doctors say that the good press vitamins get in skin care is highly overrated and I tend to agree with them. Still, many models and actresses with the most stellar skin swear by their vitamins. What to do? Educate yourself before you pop any kind of pills at all. The bottom line on vitamins and skin care seems to be this:

VITAMIN E   Once thought of as the miracle vitamin for sexuality and skin lusciousness, it's beginning to lose its allure because it doesn't always seem to perform. Those who say it speeds healing from acne scars have no real knowledge whether the skin would have healed in time, and just as well, without the E—as many doctors claim. Those who swear by the vitamin say it speeds up circulation which does nice things for the skin.

Do some research to make up your own mind. One thing's obvious, though: If you have pretty oily skin, more oil from the vitamin E capsule (that's the way it's marketed) wouldn't be so great at all. And many people report a contact dermatitis that results from using vitamin E directly on the skin.

VITAMIN A   A fat-soluble vitamin that is stored in the body, this is another very popular vitamin for skin care. Too much vitamin A can be toxic and cause hair loss and skin irritation. Literally as we go to press, the *New England Journal of Medicine* reports a new synthetic vitamin A product called isotretinoin has been found to "result in long-lasting suppression of acne." Vitamin A used topically is also called retinoic acid. Applied directly to the skin, it appears to penetrate the pores and break down the accumulated oils and bacteria that are clogging the area. Be careful with vitamin A, though: if your skin becomes reddened or irritated, discontinue its use, or check with a physician.

B VITAMINS   These are supposed to keep skin looking good, feeling pliant and blemish free, but such claims are largely unproven.

Troubletimes

You don't understand it. Weeks go by and your skin looks like Shirley Temple's and then, Zap—it's paper-bag-over-your-face time. How come? What does it? Your cleanliness routines are exactly the same as they've always been. How come a nice kid like you is being punished? The answer is that it sometimes has nothing to do with routine cleanliness or even niceness. Skin breakouts can flare up easily when one or more of the following conditions occur.

YOUR PERIOD

Menstruation can be responsible for a multitude of skin problems. Hormonal changes just before your period tend to suppress and clog the oil-producing glands and the pores through which the oil escapes. Menstruation also causes a monthly iron loss and although this is perfectly normal, the mineral deficiency sometimes does bad things even to good people's skin. Tension and particularly the condition known as PMS (Premenstrual Syndrome) can cause stress, general sluggishness in the system and bloatedness, all of which can cause an increase in oily facial secretions. Menstruating women often cut down on their exercise patterns—a big mistake for both skin and pain-free periods.

If you do have extra breakouts which you think come around the time of your monthly cycle, here's what to do: the week before your period, throw in an extra facial to compensate for the extra oiliness or any clogged condition. If you usually take three facials a week because your skin is oily, take four. If you usually take two for a relatively normal to dry skin, take three facials during that preperiod week.

Don't let added stress cause you to pick at your face or scratch it, even if you feel you *must* or you'll die. A cool cloth will soothe an angry, itchy face. If it's really terrible, perhaps your physician can prescribe something to stop the itch during this week or so.

A tip: being oily-skinned, I too am a face-toucher. To remind myself not to do it, I put a splash of cologne on the inside of my wrists and the moment I smell it, I pull my hands away from my face before they can do any damage.

YOUR VACATION

You've been saving for a year, you finally get to your exotic tropical island and you wake up on the second morning with some exotic pimples. It's not the papaya juice—it's the climate, the sea and the sun. When the climate is humid, extra perspiration and your average old skin debris tend to stick on the skin's surface, making extra cleanups during the day very important. Use your exfoliating cream more often, or even a few grains of raw oatmeal sprinkled into your cleansing lotion. A sun-screen is essential during the day. Swimming in the glorious, blue ocean waters can be romantic and exhilarating, but very drying to the skin. Fresh water carried along to the beach in a spray bottle is great for a quick salt water wash-off after your swim and even an hourly spritz for moisturizing.

Your vacation might consist of a jaunt to a wintry place where harsh winds, rain, snow or ice and a penetrating winter sun take their toll in chapped and dry skin. For especially dry skin you might try a mild urea cream like Carmol-10 which is available without a prescription and which helps the skin retain moisture. Another kind of moisturizing cream contains lactic acid, also quite effective. I suggest that you use these special creams only rarely, when your skin faces unfamiliar atmospheres as when traveling. They are not necessary for everyday use and frequent application of creams with chemical additives can do more damage than good.

When camping out on a "roughing it" vacation, even though bath water is scarce, keep an absolutely conscientious cleansing routine. You don't need water with a cleansing cream or lotion that has no perfume or soap additives. Rest assured that most cleansers billed as "sudsy," "milky," or "rinsable" are probably laden with soap and need water for rinsing.

When traveling it's a good idea to rinse much more carefully after bathing: You may be in a place where the water is hard (more minerals in it) and hard water tends to be a poor rinse for soap you may use on your face or hair. If you *must* use soap use a synthetic brand that rinses off easily and double amounts of rinse water to eradicate the thin film of soap residue that would otherwise remain. (This film not only dries the skin but can trap bacteria and dirt—anathema to good skin.)

Your mode of travel can be responsible for

skin breakouts. High altitudes, for instance, can be quite drying to skin, which is why professional models who fly a lot learn to moisturize their skin before, after and during the flight and to drink copious quantities of water during air time. A woman whose face is acclimated to pristinely pure country air may experience an inordinate amount of facial irritation from an open car window when driving through very dirty cities: She is well advised to keep the window closed and the air conditioning on at these times.

Finally, remember that the stresses of packing, meeting new people and making unfamiliar decisions as you travel can cause skin eruptions, which is why you should never take a vacation from your skin cleansing and maintenance routine.

YOUR NEW ADDITION

No, I don't mean a baby or an extra bedroom. I mean anything new that you're doing that may be contributing to a sudden facial outcry. Are you using a new cosmetic? Taking a new medication? Wearing a fabric or wool-dye that may be giving you an allergic reaction? Involved in a drastic diet change? Wearing glasses for the first time? (The glasses and your hands may be transferring oil and dirt to your face. Solution: invest in contact lenses.) Never ignore a sudden and unexpected skin assault. You may be creating it.

YOUR TENSION

There's no question that emotional stress feeds the poor-skin syndrome. Shocks to the psyche do more than jangle the nerves: They can cause tension that chokes the blood circulation, and the skin, not properly nourished by blood flow, can wither, develop lines

and crevices. Develop meditation techniques or work off tension in exercise or take a relaxing bath to relieve stress. Your skin will respond.

YOUR CONTRACEPTIVE

One of the side effects from the oral contraceptive known as The Pill can be skin problems. One of these can be an acne-type breakout. Another can be a darkening of certain parts of the skin—kind of a blotchy staining—called melasma. Exposure to the sun will make it worse. Over-the-counter bleaching preparations have started to surface which are supposed to help. Be sure that you use none containing ammoniated mercury to which many women are allergic.

YOUR FATIGUE

Chronic fatigue detests skin. When you are tired, your blood does not circulate well. Grayness of color and dark circles under the eyes are only the beginning. Toxins in the blood that are being carried away too sluggishly by the circulatory system begin to emerge on your face. Because these waste products spend too much time in the blood stream, muscle contraction becomes impaired, causing achiness and skin sag. If your skin is starting to look old when you're young, if you are plagued by constant breakouts and puffiness, you may simply be very tired.

YOUR DERMATOLOGIST

By the time you finish this book, you'll surely have a very clear idea of where I stand on most dermatologists and where I think you should stand—that is, far away. One of the troubletimes with bad skin comes precisely because you've just come home from an appointment with a dermatologist who's prescribed cortisone cream; the strong stuff you can only get with a prescription. I have never seen such oil-clogged pores in my life as I've seen on clients using prescription cortisone cream. It can also leave you with skin so fragile and thin that every vein and capillary will be visible. Many drying agents in topical acne preparations can *cause* acne if used indiscriminately. Please try my cleansing routine for a month or so before you put any medication on your face. A last word: Did you know that barbiturates can cause skin breakouts the same way steroids and vitamin B-12 in high doses can?

The Sun: Friend or Foe?

I think that the sun's had a bad press. Everywhere there are doomsayer bores warning us to stay out of the sun. These are the same bores who warned our mothers not to let us out in the night air and not to let us wash our hair every night lest it fall out. They're the ones who warned us that our organs would fall out if we didn't wear tight girdles and that reading too much would damage our eyes. Wrong, all wrong. And now, these same bores tell us that the sun is a dread enemy.

They're not altogether incorrect. Certainly, medical evidence seems to have proved that *overexposure* to sun can cause prematurely aging skin and skin cancer. I'll buy that. What I won't buy is the current hysteria against all sun exposure. It's getting so that women, concerned for their skin, wear nine layers of protection plus a hat if they happen to be dragged, kicking and screaming, to the beach. Nonsense. Sun in moderation, especially if your skin is oily and not alabaster-white, can be glorious. The rosy glow you'll get will make you look healthy, and it can also make your skin healthy when taken in small doses. Exposing the outer layer of skin to the sun stimulates cell growth which results in a peeling process that helps keep pores open— and less vulnerable to oil clog or infection. The sun, again in small doses, definitely helps heal the crusty, flaky blotches of the skin condition known as psoriasis. It dries up plain old pimples. It helps tense muscles to loosen. It relaxes. It draws blood to the surface, improving circulation which in turn moves those impurities in the blood stream up and out. The sun's swell. Still, there are precautions you should use to avoid an overaccumulation of ultraviolet rays which can be disease-producing and aging. I tell my clients to wear any one or more of the following, depending on the vulnerability of their skin:

* a moisturizer;
* a makeup base through which the sun *will* penetrate, giving a nice, rosy tone instead of a true tan;
* a sun block.

True sun blocks should contain PABA (para-aminobenzoic acid) which actually absorbs the ultraviolet rays of the sun. If you tend to burn easily, apply your sun block again after swimming and stay relatively covered up in the sun's strongest moments— between 11 A.M. and 2 P.M. And remember that even on a hazy day, the sun is shining through on you. But again, the word is moderation.

If you're not a Summer Crazy who sits with a torture reflector, if you don't consider the sun a religious experience, don't let the bores take its nurturing rays completely away.

On the slim chance that you just might overdo it, despite all these wise words, here are two immediate sunburn-pain relievers.

TANNIC ACID SOOTHER   Plain tea bags allowed to steep in a cup of boiling water and then cool are wonderfully soothing pats on a sunburned face. Dip the bags into the cooled tea and softly tap your face with them for about ten minutes. Blot dry with soft cloth.

BAKING SODA PAIN BLITZ   Equal parts of baking soda and warm water, patted on and left for half an hour is helpful.

You Are What You Eat—You Look It, Too!

Skin care is related to total health and total health is very much dependent on what goes in your mouth. It's a definite interconnected cycle, and if you want to have good skin you cannot ignore diet. For instance, poor diet often brings about gastrointestinal problems which in turn create loose, hanging and wrinkled skin; broken blood vessels; rashes; itchy, scaly, puffy skin. Infections, which become more easily contracted when nutritional strength is undermined, can create inflamed hair follicles on the skin, boils, pimples, cracked lips—it's too depressing to go on.

What's more, all those bogus creams with placentas, vitamins, hormones and herb extracts added don't really do any good at all for your face because the goodness has to come from *inside* the body to the outside skin—not the other way around. Most exotic substances added in facial creams simply don't penetrate beyond the superficial layer of skin.

Shining, soft, healthy skin has to eat and what *it* eats are the beneficial by-products of what *you* eat. Not long ago, scientists were crazed over the Case of the Orange Man. Seems this guy came to his doctor with orange skin and nobody could find what was causing it. He wasn't sick, he wasn't hallucinating; he was just orange. It took only one commonsense doctor to ask the right questions and figure the whole thing out: It seems the Orange Man just loved raw carrots and ate at least ten a day. His skin was trying to tell him something. So, the well-being of your body, your mind, your whole digestive system shows in your skin.

Since this is not a diet book, and I am not concerned with weight loss or gain properties of food, I simply offer you seven nutritional shortcuts to health, and thereby to skin beauty. The seven tips are culled from the commonsense advice of experts and doctors whom I respect—and who seem to have the best-looking skin in town.

✻ Don't be a food stick-in-the-mud. The trick to good health is to eat a *variety* of different foods and to know what's in each. Most foods are really many foods. Sure, protein is good for your skin, but don't be misled into thinking that if meat is protein, a lot of meat must be good for your skin. Hamburger alone is two-thirds fat, and all that fat clogs pores as well as blood vessels! Milk contains calcium, sure, but also a lot of fat, carbohydrates, vitamins A and D, riboflavin and phosphorus.

✻ Although this may seem heretical, I say don't be scared off by nutrition bullies. Everything that's not wonderful for you will not kill you either and moderation is the key word. People who are neurotic about what they must *not* eat under pain of death, cancer or pimples are generally tense people, and you know what tenseness does to the skin's oil production. Take the cholesterol-obsessed. Cholesterol will surely be the end of you, they smugly say. But science, as we note several times in this book, changes its mind regularly and now the scientists are saying that high blood cholesterol levels are not a function of the food you eat, after all. Take salt. It's not the healthiest thing in the world, but a little drop won't make your skin or the rest of you fall apart. A good idea is to use the salt that doesn't contain iodine instead of the familiar iodized stuff because iodine is a mineral that aggravates pimples and acne. So be moderate in all food things, but not fanatic.

* Sugar doesn't give you pimples, but it can give you a fat face. It undermines health by causing teeth to decay; it's also a factor in low blood-sugar levels because the body's insulin production is over-stimulated, resulting in the liver and muscles drawing too much from sugar from the blood (a vicious cycle). Sugar's not your best friend, but who doesn't need an occasional Milky Way? I sure do.

* Be responsible for your own diet and don't leave it all to Dr. Stillman, Dr. Atkins or the Scarsdale Doctor—you know what happened to him! Your body and your skin will tell you if you're on the right track with foods. Do you have energy, fewer colds and blemishes, fewer depressions with five small meals a day rather than three large ones? Stick to the five. Do salads make you crave more substantial foods? Salads are not your best food choice then, no matter what the models say. Does a twenty-four-hour fast every couple of weeks or so make you feel rejuvenated? Do it! Try to eat lean meats, chicken, veal, fish as often as possible; try to eat fresh fruits and vegetables—ah, you *know* all the rules already. The trick is to use your common sense. What makes you feel good and look good is probably the food pattern that's preordained for your particular chemical balance. Trust yourself and throw out all the diet books.

* Try the natural moisturizers. To moisturize from the inside out there are three natural moisturizers: lactic acid, found in milk and other dairy products; malic acid, found in apples; and citric acid, found in grapefruit, lemons and oranges. A diet rich in these agents seems to polish the skin by helping the outer layers to peel off easily without flaking and clogging the pores.

* Certain foods can cause skin problems. The so-called "blushing foods"—hot, peppery, spicy substances—can permanently enlarge the capillaries and give you a roughened, reddened look. Dry skin is particularly susceptible to this problem. Too much caffeine and alcohol can produce the same results and dry out the skin as well. Iodine and bromide-rich foods like shellfish, seaweed or kelp can cause or worsen acne. Suddenly becoming a vegetarian can cause pallor because you've cut out the best absorbed forms of iron, found in meat, chicken and fish. Salt causes your body to retain water and make your skin look puffy and bloated.

* Although in many ways you are what you eat, your pimples are not what they are because you eat chocolate, sweets or fried foods. Hershey Bars are not magically swept from the mouth to the blood stream. The skin's oil is manufactured by local oil glands and the amount given off doesn't reflect diet. Excess oil clogging the pores comes from inside; it is related to hormonal activity and inheritance rather than gluttony.

Annoyances, Embarrassments, Protuberances and Other Skin-Uglies

The *things* that can come out of that facial skin! Take, for instance,

HAIR Glamorous, gorgeous silver hair, raven hair, auburn hair, chestnut hair, golden hair—it all makes a woman more glorious; except when it's over her lip. Facial hair, despite the good press that the swarthy beauties of Latin America get, is not received terrifically well here in America. In fact, some of the most ardent feminists get rid of their mustaches—if they have them. So should you. But how?

Wax it, that's how. It's really the best way. A cream or chemical depilatory cannot get as deep down and so only removes the surface hair, which means it grows back posthaste. And then again, certain products cause irritation and redness, especially if they've been hanging around the house too long. Bleaching doesn't remove hair; it's always still there and sometimes more obvious than ever because instead of being just dark, it's positively glowing with platinum good health. And if you shave your face, you deserve what you get—five o'clock shadow. Electrolysis is generally safe but it's costly, painful and the hair can sometimes grow back. It has also been known to leave perfect, round little holes in the face of those treated by unskilled operators.

Waxing pulls the hair out from the root so it leaves a long-lasting, smooth, clean surface. Although you can opt to have your face (and arms and legs and bikini-line) waxed in a beauty salon, there's no earthly reason why you can't do it yourself at home, more cheaply and easily.

This is how you wax. You should buy, in any beauty supply store, the cheapest facial wax you can find (Zip is good). Spending a whole lot of money on perfumed, beautifully boxed wax that will end up in the garbage with a whole lot of little hairs stuck to it is the worst conspicuous consumption there is.

1. Clean your face thoroughly, dry it, and put a layer of talcum powder between your skin and the wax for easy removal.

2. Apply the wax first to one side of the upper lip only, making sure to cover all the facial hair on that side. Let harden thoroughly.

3. With one hand hold the skin on the other side of the lip firmly; with your free hand, pull the wax off in one firm pull (if you do it slowly, it's the Hot Wax Torture). Press the pad of your finger directly over the waxed area and apply pressure for a minute. This soothes and helps prevent water blisters from building up. Now, do other side of the lip the same way.

The waxing should last about a month.

You can do your chin, the nape of your neck (if you have short hair) and your sideburns and hairline if they get scraggly. If you do your hairline, *keep* it looking neat to avoid the five o'clock temple look. Remember: wait till the wax hardens fully before pulling it off.

A word of caution: if you are prone to ingrown hairs, waxing may be difficult.

PERSPIRATION   We all know that it's healthy to perspire, but it does nasty things to your confidence and your makeup when your whole face is awash in gleaming sweat. Antiperspirants (different from deodorants) can help to control the perspiration that comes under your arms, but the face is another story since you can't put Secret on your upper lip. Sometimes it helps to put a light dusting of plain bicarbonate of soda under your foundation if you know you perspire heavily and you want your makeup to stay matte. It's particularly important for you to use powder when you make up, both to set the color and to discourage facial perspiration. Dressing coolly, ducking into a bathroom to apply cold water to your wrists and the back of your neck as often as possible and wearing a light, cool cologne all help to keep body temperature and perspiration down. Finally, there's nothing like occlusive face junk—excess oils, very heavy creams and oil-based foundations—to clog facial pores and cause bacterial infections from the stopped-up perspiration. Something good about aging: sweat glands decrease in size due to hormone changes and perspiration slows.

ROTTEN ROSACEA Rosacea is a disease of the oil glands expressed by severe inflammation and infection on the face. It looks like teenage acne: Because of the blood vessel enlargement which occurs with the excess oil produced, the skin where the lesions appear looks unpleasantly red. Diet helps. Forgo spices, coffee, tea, milk and alcohol. Sometimes antibiotics help but try some Sulforcin lotion on your own before you even see a doctor. Makeup doesn't add to the problem so try to mask the red nose as best you can. Sometimes, emotional highs and lows and exposure to extreme conditions of weather can bring on an attack of rosacea, and then, perhaps, a tranquilizer might be in order—doctor prescribed, of course. Cursing helps a lot.

TINY, BROKEN CAPILLARIES They're broken blood vessels from too much wine drinking or pimple squeezing. Electric needles applied by a doctor can coagulate the blood and make the capillaries whiten.

MOLES These are pigmented growths on the skin that can be removed painlessly and quickly by a plastic surgeon or a very skilled dermatologist. Once gone, you're generally rid of them for good.

WARTS Caused by a virus, they can appear and disappear no matter how many times you have them removed. Physicians use painless acid, surgery, ultrasonics and freezing with liquid nitrogen to take them off—all in an effort to banish the miseries. When you have moles or warts on your face, it's often a very good idea to see a plastic surgeon rather than a dermatologist. The former will give you better odds on getting rid of the complaint without facial scarring.

Sensitive Skin, Allergic Skin

It doesn't help to buy products with a "hypoallergenic" label, because hypoallergenic means almost nothing. The only thing it legally implies is that the manufacturer has found the product doesn't irritate one kind of condition or person, to the exclusion of all else. Perhaps, for instance, the product was tested on guinea pigs or mice. And the pigs and mice came out marvelously clear-skinned. Well, that's super news for the pigs and mice and the manufacturer can say the product is hypoallergenic. Or "allergy" tested. Or "dermatologist" tested. That doesn't mean *you* can't get warts, bumps or itches. In plain language, you can definitely be allergic to any hypoallergenic product. Here is a tip sheet of good and bad bets for easily irritated skin.

GOOD BETS

* White sheets. Heavily patterned or dyed sheets have dyes that may irritate. They also lose softness more quickly.
* Cosmetics or skin products with *no* alcohol or perfume added.
* Total sunblocks when you're outside in summer and also on cold, windy winter days; the best 100 percent sunblock is zinc oxide.
* Eye creams (nonperfumed) are a necessity for you. Pat onto this extremely delicate area very gently.
* Buy cosmetics in small sizes to avoid spoilage. Close them tightly and keep in closed, cool cabinets. Heat can change their composition and cause them to become irritants.
* Use 100 percent cotton balls or Coets on your face—no synthetic puffs.
* Wash new sheets or blouses before use to soften the fabric and at least partially get rid of any irritating starches and other preservatives.
* If you *must* use perfume, spray it on clothing; keep it away from the neck.

* If the color in lipstick seems to irritate your lips coat them first with a clear gloss and then brush on color. I prefer an aloe gloss product.

* Certain jewelry contains nickel which is a well known irritant. Avoid it. Tell your lover you can only deal with pure gold or silver.

BAD BETS

* Cosmetics with perfumes are bad news. You can check any cosmetic to see if it will "get you" by rubbing some on your wrist and leaving it there for twenty-four hours. If you get an itchy, red or swollen wrist, imagine what your face will look like.

* Steaming your face in those medieval facial torture chambers will almost certainly blow it up. Hot baths, ice water extremes are irritating to sensitive skin.

* Sun lamps are out. Ultraviolet rays *hate* allergic skin.

* Grainy cleansers, scrubby brushes.

* Going out in *any* weather without a moisturizer.

* Eye liner on the inside rim of your eye can irritate very sensitive skin.

* Soap.

* Hair dye.

* Polluted air, including smoke-filled rooms.

3 *

Facing Front: Makeup

SINCE TIME IMMEMORIAL, women have been coloring their faces. It must be an important human need—this desire to create prettiness from paint—and those who would scoff at the "frivolity" of the need would make terrible social scientists. Cro-Magnon woman put daubs of clay on her prehistoric features to give them *flaunt*—and rest assured, her caveman admirers approved. Cleopatra, Jezebel, Nefertiti, witch doctors, rich doctors all did it. Ophelia puts a dab or so of lipstick on her tragic mouth— even if Hamlet says she shouldn't. The ancient Egyptians wouldn't be caught embalmed without their pots of black kohl. Nero's Roman beauties whitened their cheeks with chalk and used barley powder to camouflage their classic Roman pimples. Even the Puritan maidens who were expressly forbidden by their religion to use makeup (probably on the theory that anything that good-looking must be bad) were not above pinching their virtuous cheeks to raise a bit of color.

So, although times change and power rests in different hands, the urge to look more beautiful—to make an impression on others with makeup—never does change. Gloria Steinem wears blusher. I guarantee it. So does my mother. So does my grandmother, as you'll see elsewhere in this book. The "naturalists" who inveigh heavily against makeup are waging a losing battle. Women can look natural *and* can look gorgeous. Historically, emotionally, practically—looking pretty is as much a desired part of a woman's life as independence, nurturing and creativity. And makeup, carefully, artfully applied, makes you look prettier. It really does . . .

Makeup does away with the age distinctions that have been referred to by one of my clients as youth, middle age and gee, you look great. With makeup, everyone at every age can *really* look great. You may hear your man say he hates makeup on women, but if you look terrific, he'll pretend not to notice it.

Too many heavy-hype makeup artists would have you believe that there's something mysterious about makeup application. The theory that each face is so unique that only an artist working on *your* particular face could show you how to make it up beautifully is nothing more than over-brag. What's more, even worse than over-brag, is

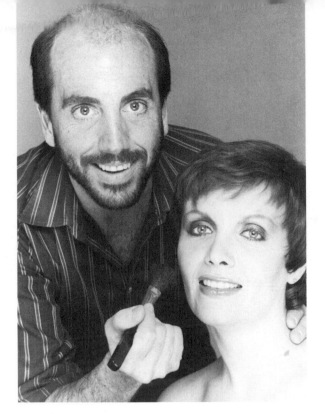

JEFFREY BRUCE
with MAUREEN McGOVERN.

the overkill theory, which rests in the delusion that a woman needs endless rainbows of color and cream variations to keep her looking terrific. Just this year, one major cosmetics company's newest shiny brochure boasts that it offers lipsticks in 269 landmark colors, 70 glosses and 156 nail enamels. Now that, my friends, is overkill.

All a woman ever *really* needs is one clear gloss that can be applied with any lipstick for a translucent shine; at most two or three glosses in a copper, pink or coral to subtly change the look of the one or two lipsticks in your makeup cabinet. Any woman who is noted for wearing 269 landmark colors is an extreme woman, to say the least. Ditto for nail enamel.

And I hate to tell you, your face is not so unique. You have two eyes, one nose and one mouth like everyone else and in basically the same arrangement. With some variations, of course, in color and technique, your basic makeup procedures essentially should be not so very different from your best friend's. Once you learn the techniques, buy the basic products (very few of them, at that) and have perhaps one or two professional make ups, you should do wonderfully with your own face—without the artist who thinks he's indispensable in your life. You do not need that hot orange or passion purple lipstick that's been sitting in your makeup cabinet for a year. You do not need it because it's ugly. And you had doubts about it when you bought it—right? You don't need the eleven brushes that take up too much room. It's not that you don't need makeup. You do. And you probably need more than you've been used to applying, even though the faddists say less. What you need is fewer products, more artfully applied—and that should give you the understated, exquisite look you've always admired on certain women. Make no mistake: The understated look is still a very definite statement. It requires the right products and a full and thoughtful application. The natural look doesn't come from avocado facials or pressed berries. It comes from makeup—careful and integrated makeup—that's quite simple to learn. What follows is a list of all the makeup products you'll ever need.

All the Makeup Products You Ever Need

You do not need thirty-nine lipsticks. You do not need nine eye shadows. Simplify your life and your makeup cabinet. All you have to do is:

Choose a day when you have an hour to kill. Take *everything* out of your makeup cabinet. If you've had any product longer

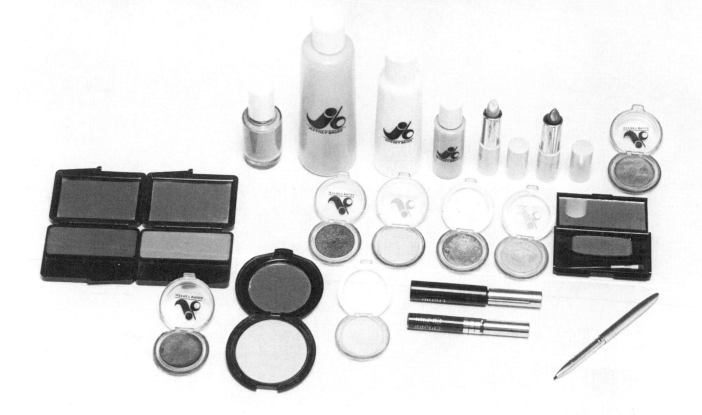

than one year, throw it out. Now. If you have any products that are missing lids, covers or other integral parts, throw them out. Now. Be ruthless. Sponge out your makeup cabinet and put back only the following makeup— anything more is conspicuous consumption; the tools you need will follow.

PRODUCTS YOU NEED

1. *Lipsticks*—2 or 3: more is extravagant. Lip glosses can temper a lipstick color to change its look, so if you have a couple of lipsticks and two or three glosses, that's plenty.
2. *Lip Glosses*—4: copper, pink, coral, clear.
3. *Foundation*—1: in cream form if you need more coverage or in liquid form for less coverage. Throw out the too light or too dark foundations that came as "gifts" with your last makeup purchase. Your foundation should only be in a shade that's a trifle lighter than your skin. And you don't have to change it in the wintertime: Makeup doesn't keep you warm.

4. *Blusher*—1: in a soft, rosy shade to simulate a real blush.
5. *Contour*—1: in a rusty, brownish shade.
6. *Cream Rouge*—1: in a soft red, pink or coral—whichever is closest to your own blushing color.
7. *Liquid Under-eye Concealer*—1.
8. *Translucent Powder*—1 box.
9. *Eye Shadows*—4: See the Guide to Your Best Colors to determine the colors that are best for you. With four shadows, you can make many different looks, depending on where you put the shadows. Experiment with many colors to see what different combinations can do for you.
10. *Eyeliner Crayon*—1: in a charcoal grey or soft brown.
11. *Brush-on Brow Powder*—1 box, or 1 sharp brown crayon: in a shade that matches your natural brows. You need a small, wedge-shaped brush for the brow powder.
12. *Lip Liner Pencil*—1.
13. *Shadow Seal*—1: to be applied before the eye shadow color: This seals the color onto the lid. If you have a light, whitish eye-shadow powder, this will do just fine.

14. *Moisturizer:* to help the makeup slide on and blend easily, and to keep it from being absorbed into the skin.
15. *Black Mascara Wand.*

Remember to test. If you don't test your makeup, you have no idea what to expect because every product looks different in the container from the way it does on your skin. Test foundations from the sample bottles on your *face,* not on your wrist.

That's it for the makeup.

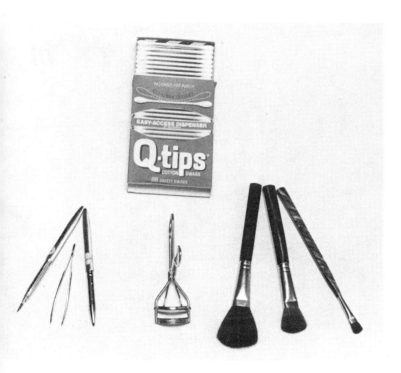

TOOLS OF THE TRADE

Sable Brushes—3: one for eye shadow, one for contour, one for powder and blusher. If you use *good* brushes, the powders will not adhere to the bristle and will come off with a blow.
Lip-Color Brush—1.
Eyelash Curler—1.
Tweezers—1.

Q-Tips—1 box, for applying concealer, dotting on makeup, smudging eyeliner, removing mistakes—a million uses!

SPECIAL TIPS

* Don't buy large sizes. The longer you keep a product, the better chance it has of drying out, becoming contaminated, losing potency. If you must buy a large size, transfer into several smaller containers and keep all tightly closed and stored in a cool place.

* If a cream changes consistency or if any product develops an odor, throw it out.

* Always wash hands before (and even while) you apply makeup. Sometimes the "allergic" reaction you think comes from a makeup comes from dirty hands which have contaminated it.

* Don't assume you are not allergic to a cosmetic just because you have not been in the past. Allergies can develop after years of successfully using a product. If in doubt about a sensitivity or allergy, because of a sudden reaction, try changing your usual brand of cosmetic to see what happens.

It's one thing to buy makeup and quite another to apply it properly. What follows is the basic makeup routine I teach my clients. The niceties and the fine points will come later.

Morning Premakeup Routine

THE FACE WASH

You don't need anything as concentrated as a regular skin cleanser in the morning because you've taken your makeup off the night before with the cleanser. *Haven't you?* All you have to do then is clean and wake up your skin. There are many ways of doing this without soap, which is the poorest choice of all. For normal to dry skin, I use a light cleanser called a Liqui-Facial. It's non-alkaline and has no lanolin which tends to dry skin and clog pores. Oily skin would do better with a slightly lemon cleanser which is more acidic and gets the pores cleansed and closed without creating surface dryness. You use the light cleansers the same way you use soap and water: lather up, lightly massage, rinse off.

THE FRESHENER

A freshener wakes up the skin and also helps to remove any dirt or cream left by the face wash. I use a product without perfumes or alcohol but with lime juice which has been substituted for the alcohol in most fresheners. Pat it on with a Coet or cotton ball and allow to dry for a few seconds.

THE DERMAL-FEEDER MOISTURIZER

The purpose of a moisturizer is to seal in moisture, that's why it's best applied over damp skin. This prevents the lines that *would* come from too-dry skin from appearing and it also softens the lines you already have. It cannot prevent the wrinkling that is your birthright. I use a special cream called a dermal-feeder because it is created from aloe and collagen. It's the protein fibers known as collagen that give strength and elasticity to your skin, and as you age the body loses some of the moisture that helps the collagen fibers stay woven together like interconnected fingers. When the moisture starts to escape, the collagen separates and wrinkles and lines begin to appear on the skin's surface. The moisturizer seals in more moisture, restores some of the collagen to the skin and also provides a lubricating base that will help your foundation blend easily over the skin's surface. Another function of the moisturizer is to prevent the foundation base from being absorbed into the skin. Now, you do not have to use an aloe and collagen dermal-feeder moisturizer, but be very sure that the product you use is not heavy with oils that just sit there on top of your skin clogging the pores instead of being light enough to allow the skin to absorb moisture and nourishment.

THE JEFFREY BRUCE MAKEUP

Steady yourself with a glass of champagne, which helps enormously if you make terrible mistakes. Your makeup, this first time, may take close to an hour to apply. Tomorrow, I promise you, it will take fifteen minutes. As I go through the directions, keep in mind that it is my own aloe-based products that I keep referring to, but you may substitute any of my own line with a similar product from another manufacturer. In order of their appearance, here are the proper steps to a wonderful makeup.

PRELUDE

First things first. Get to know your face. Really know it. Touch it to feel the skin texture, the bones, the hollows. See where the skin is taut and where it will need to be "tightened up" with color. Look at your face as if it is the first time you are seeing it: That's not easy to do. Most women have a funny mirror inside their real mirror: They see what they believe themselves to be, and that can either be Cinderella or Quasimodo. Look at your real self, the eye overhang, the lines, the dark circles. See the potential— good nose? great bones?—but don't block out the reality, what has to be improved with makeup.

Now, you're ready to start.

THE MAKEUP BASE

The purpose of makeup base, or foundation, is to equalize the pigment of skin, *not* to give it color despite what you've read up till now. This foundation should be a color that's a half-shade *lighter* than your own complexion, never darker. Darkness stains blemishes while the lighter foundation will conceal problems. Dot the foundation on over your face, lips (this protects lipstick from turning a darker shade on your mouth) and down to the jawline. Quickly blend the color upward and downward with your fingertips (no, this won't make facial muscles sag) using light, circular, buff-and-polish movements. Liquid base (used when you need minimal coverage) should be applied with a Q-Tip, and cream base (for maximum coverage on ruddy, oily or blemished complexions) should be applied with fingertips. Thin out fluid as you near the jawline; blend color over the jawline but not on the neck, to avoid stains on your clothing. Never use a sponge to apply foundation: It eats up more than it delivers. If you're doubtful about this, check out your sink when you wash a makeup sponge.

Foundation also comes in gels (light, transparent coverage), foams (very light coverage), and cakes (very heavy, artificial coverage—they're awful!).

*

Note: Never try to put cheek color on your face without first putting on a foundation. It will look blotchy as hell and be very irritating to your skin. Foundation, like moisturizer, serves a protective function as well as evening your complexion. The worst skin I ever see is on women who wear no makeup at all. The next worst skin is on women who wear rouge, blusher and contour without a foundation base.

If you don't already have your own favorite foundation, you might consider these.

* Borghese Lumina (normal to dry skin, a medium coverage)
* Chanel Teint Naturel Liquid (gives maximum coverage, use a very little)
* Clinique Balanced Base (for normal–oily skin)

Corrective work comes next, just before color is added to the face.

THE MAKEUP BASE

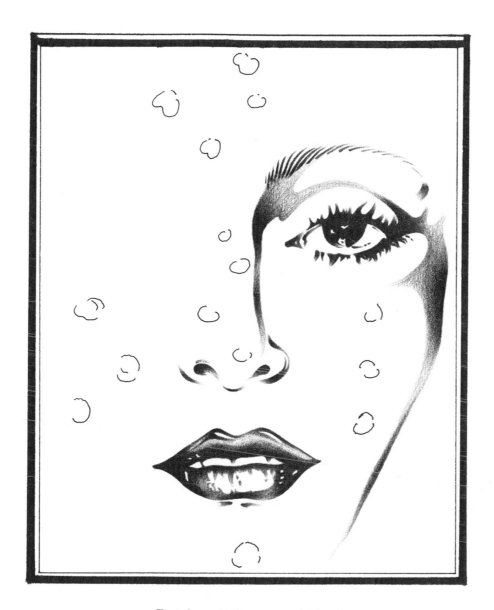

Dot foundation on and blend.

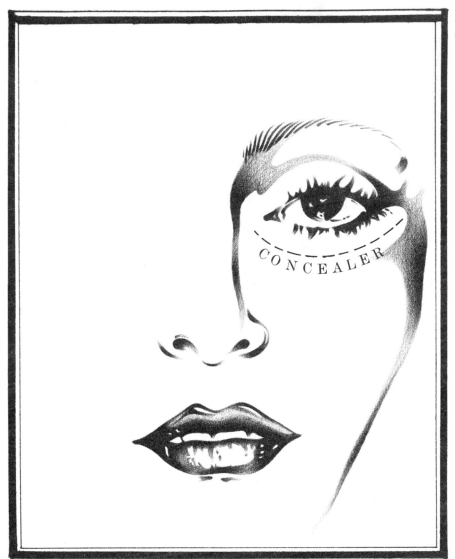

Dot concealer only on
line of demarcation
and blend.

Concealer should be in the form of a light beige liquid, not a cream or cake, so it won't congeal inside the facial lines. Apply it in small dots directly onto the line of demarcation you wish to hide. Don't spread it on the puffy part of the under-eye or bring it up to your lower lashes because then you will closely resemble a raccoon. Concealer is also used on any blemishes or dark spots on your face. Blend in the concealing liquid with your fingertips. On Stage puts out a good concealer.

Note: Many makeup artists put the concealer on *before* the foundation base. I could never understand why. If you do it their way, the concealer will swim away as soon as you blend in the foundation.

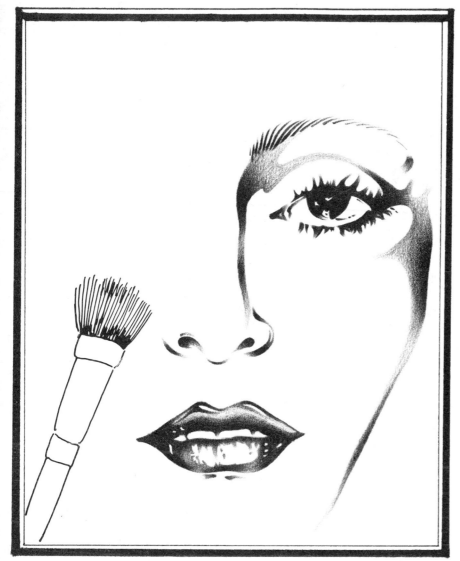

Lightly brush your face with translucent powder.

It's time for the first dusting of powder. Many women fear that powder will give a dry, aged, whitefaced clown look, but a translucent powder only sets makeup and obliterates shine (one of my biggest hates). It does not add color, and if carefully and lightly applied it will surely not add pastiness. A moist, dewy look is delightful; a shining, oily look is not, and translucent powder can make the difference. I powder with a large, flat sable brush which can be bought at cosmetic counters or in any good supply house. It's expensive, but don't try to save money here.

A good brush can be used forever and washed in the top tray of the dishwasher (remove it before the dry cycle). When you use a good sable brush, it doesn't leave little black hairs on your face, nor does it make heavy applications. It merely softly sets, smooths, blends. A good brush is the whole secret of blending. I could not do without it.

Translucent powders come in loose box form or pressed compact form. You might try the products of Chanel, Lancôme or Elizabeth Arden.

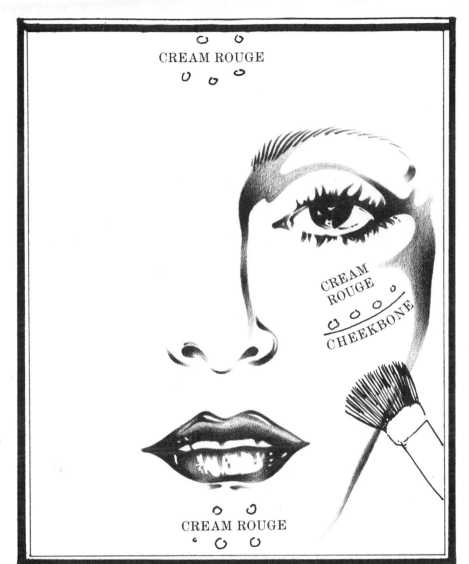

CREAM ROUGE

CREAM ROUGE

CHEEKBONE

CREAM ROUGE

Brush contour under cheekbone.

Dot cream rouge over cheekbone and on chin and forehead. Blend.

Powder over rouge with blusher.

One of the most frequent questions I'm asked is, ''How do I get that classic cheekbone line?'' The answer is with *powdered* contour. It helps to chisel out high cheekbones and give your face interest and character. Contour goes *under* the cheekbone, not on or near the jawline. Sucking in your cheeks, despite the common myth, will not show you the proper place to contour.

Touch your fingers to the hard bones on your cheeks—that's the cheekbone. Now, feel underneath—that's musculature. The contour goes in that hollow and is blended outward from the middle of the cheek to the hairline in an upward slant. Don't stop before the hairline, and don't make the hairline area darker than the rest. Apply the powdered contour with a flat-end brush and blend carefully. Contour should be a rich brown-rust shade.

Contour powder can make double chins, wide noses, long noses, sagging necks and other problems less obvious. You might try Biba's contour powder.

THE COLOR

Color comes after the contour. The color is comprised of cream rouge *and* powder blusher: If you use just one and not the other, you'll end up with disappearing color in half an hour. Dot the cream rouge *on* the cheekbones, following the line of the contour. Dot a bit on the chin and forehead, also. The color should simulate a natural blush, and when you blush you don't do it in two perfect stripes. Blend the dots evenly to meld with the contour: There should never be a line where the rouge ends and the contour begins. Now, take a brush and lightly powder over the cream rouge with blusher. That sets the color. It will last and last.

Cheek color should never scream; it should be a softened red or pink or coral. *Never* little, round, Raggedy Ann circles. *Never* lightning jags. *Never* clown spots. Always, *always* soft; muted; blended. Then, with your big flat brush, powder again with translucent powder over the whole makeup to set and give a matte finish.

Alexandra de Markoff puts out a nice blusher and I like Borghese Lumina cream rouge.

THE EYES

They can be made hauntingly beautiful and can seize the attention and imagination like no other feature. First—

SHADOW SEAL This is a light, white powder which I put on the lids of the eyes before any eye shadow is applied. It is my secret weapon to prevent oil from collecting in the crease of the lid. It seals the powder eye shadows on firmly. Any white or beige eye shadow can be used as a shadow seal.

BROWS There's nothing worse than a painted line trying to pass for an eyebrow.

Ideally, brow color should come in pressed powder form and be applied with a small, slanted, wedge-shaped brush. The point on the wedge is used to draw in tiny extra hairs to fill in any bald spots on the skin. Remember—you're not coloring brow hairs, you're coloring the skin in between. If you must use a pencil, make sure it's very sharp.

Brow color ought to come in either blond, light brown, charcoal grey or auburn to match your own brow color. One is all you'll ever need. Feather in the brow color lightly where there are no hairs. Brows should be seen and not heard: No one wants his attention drawn to your eyebrows—it's your eyes he's interested in. Estēe Lauder puts out an excellent brow powder.

EYE SHADOWS Here, I have the most fun. I use four shadows on almost every woman and the colors depend not on eye color but on skin and hair color and what she's wearing. Eye shadow that matches your eyes will draw attention away from them. The idea is to complement eye color! The brush used for shadows (and shadows should always be in powder, not cream form) is a small fluff brush. Never use a sponge on your eyes, you'll have too little control.

✳ *The first shadow* is a highlighting color that goes under the brow and meets the lid color. It creates space and interest and is in a lighter shade than the lid color.

✳ *The second shadow* is the primary color that goes on the lid. It accentuates the iris color—doesn't match it—and disguises puffiness or lid overhang. It's in a quiet, muted shade.

✳ *The third shadow* is swept on the outer corner of the eye in a flare from the upper lash-line to the brow-line. It usually starts about the middle of the lash-line and is car-

FOUR EYE SHADOWS AND MASCARA

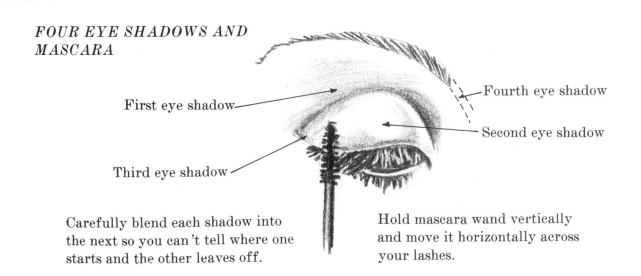

First eye shadow

Fourth eye shadow

Second eye shadow

Third eye shadow

Carefully blend each shadow into the next so you can't tell where one starts and the other leaves off.

Hold mascara wand vertically and move it horizontally across your lashes.

---

ried out to the end of the brow. It widens the eye, opens the eye, separates the two eyes and must be finely blended into the other shadows. It might pick up the color of something you're wearing or be a tint of your iris shade.

* *The fourth shadow* (the last one) is brushed on from the bridge-bone of the nose to the start of the eyebrow—right in that inner corner. It gives depth and also enlarges the eye. It's in a muted shade.

The color tip to remember is this: *lightness brings out, darkness hides.* The lightest shadows go under the brow to bring out and exaggerate the width and space around the eye and the darker shadows go on the lid of the eye, especially along the crease, to mute any eye overhang or drooping awnings.

To apply eye shadow: Brush the *first shadow* under the eyebrow to meet the lid. Next, to open up the eyes, apply the *second shadow* on the lid and blend it into the first shadow. The first shadow should end approximately at the crease of the eye, where the darker second shadow begins. With tiny, buffing brush strokes, apply the *third shadow* on a diagonal from the middle of the lash-line to the end of the brow, filling in the outer quarter of the eye in a flaring, triangular shape.

Working on a diagonal instead of coloring in neat, straight layers gives the eyes a natural and larger look. This third shadow can also be applied under the lower lashes in a *thin* line from the center of the lower lash-line to the outer corner of the eye, and then gently smudged. The *fourth and last shadow* is gently brushed on in a muted line connecting the bridge of the nose with the start of the brow and blended softly in that inner corner of the eye.

One should never be able to really see a line of demarcation where one shadow begins and another leaves off: They all should be softly blended together. It takes time to get the procedure down pat. Play with it often, till you find it comes naturally. Below are some of the eye shadow powders I've found to have clear color and staying power.

* Alexandra de Markoff
* Estée Lauder Pressed Eyelid Shadow
* Halston
* Lancôme Maquiriche CremePowder EyeColour
* Ultima II (available in duos, trios or foursomes)

Note: Many eye shadows come with silly little sponge applicators which should be discarded and a small, soft brush substituted.

EYELINERS   Almost always use a crayon instead of a liquid eyeliner; it's much softer looking and can be softly smudged. (The exception is when you are applying false eyelashes.) I use a frozen aloe crayon which is very smooth; it doesn't pull at the eye skin and it's completely nonallergic, so people who wear contacts don't have to worry about crayon getting into the inner tear duct and irritating the eye.

Draw a soft line just where there are lashes and then softly blend it with your fingertip. *Never* extend the crayon line beyond the lashes, in wings heading toward the stratosphere. Eyeliner is applied above the line of the upper lashes (there should never be a space between the lash-line and the crayon line) and below the line of the lower lashes. Sometimes, it's applied *in* the lower rim of the eye (the wet ledge) to make the whites seem whiter. Chanel's eye crayon is absolutely superb, in my judgment.

MASCARA   Loads of it and always in black, please! Everyone knows you're wearing mascara and you're allowed to be dramatic here, when the key word is subtle everywhere else. Before you apply mascara, curl your eyelashes with the eyelash curler. If you do it after the mascara is applied half your lashes will come out when you remove the curler.

Now pay attention: I've found a way to apply mascara that seems to make lashes look thicker and longer. Hold your mascara wand vertically, not horizontally as you've been taught. With the tip of the wand, and from left to right, apply the mascara horizontally from the lashes in the corner of the eye to the outer lashes. It gives a lovely, thick look without clotting and clumping. Do the bottom lashes the same way, but don't use quite as much mascara. If your eyelashes are clotted with mascara, an old toothbrush does wonders to even them out. Time for blending with more loose powder and the finishing brush; loosely pat your whole face and nose to set your makeup. One of the best mascaras around comes from Lancôme.

EYELINER

Lash-line: Apply crayon *over* line and smudge.

Inner ledge of eye

Lash-line: Apply crayon *under* line and gently smudge.

Crayon line should meld with lash-line; there should never be any space in between.

Crayon can be applied inside lower ledge of eye.

THE LIPS

Only one color is ever appropriate for lip liner and that is burgundy, which is an intensification of your own lip color and can be used with any lipstick color. With tiny strokes, outline the lips. If you have a thin or a too-full mouth that needs some cosmetic redesigning, here's what you do: Look closely at your lips in the mirror. There is a clear pigmented line of demarcation on each lip but then, above and below each lip, there's another, much paler lip-line. If you need to make your mouth fuller, follow the outline of the outer lip-line as you line your lips. If you wish to make your mouth less full, you'll follow the outline of the inner, more definite lip-line. The purpose of lip liner is twofold: to outline the lips and to prevent the lipstick from bleeding outside of the lip-line into those tiny age lines so many women tend to develop. Carefully blend the lip liner into the lip color so you don't have an artificial "coloring book" line around your lips. Make sure you've smoothed foundation base and a light dusting of powder on your lips before you line and color them. This evens the pigment and gives staying power to the lipstick.

Now, here's the secret of the most luscious lips in town: Take your lip brush and dip it into some clear gloss. Now, dip it into the lip color you've chosen. Paint the combined gloss/color inside the outlined lips to give a moist, translucent glow to your mouth. Most women just glop the clear gloss thickly onto the lip after the color and that makes a mouth that looks like you can go ice skating on it—or else one that's had a coat of polyurethane applied.

If you should inadvertently buy a lipstick that's dry and has no slip, return it! If cosmetics are inferior, you should always return them. Below are listed some manufacturers

Pale outer lip-line (outline here)

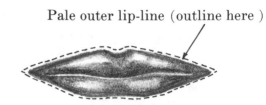

Pale inner lip-line (outline here)

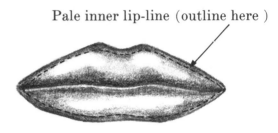

of lipsticks which I've found consistently creamy and longer lasting.

> Chanel
> Diane Von Furstenberg
> Frances Denney
> Ultima II

Note: Many lipsticks are *outrageously* priced today, with some costing $13.50 (Yves Saint Laurent) or more. Some of the factors that may be included in a good lipstick are a built-in sunscreen, creaminess, and long-lasting action.

And that's it for a perfect makeup! You're ready to meet the world. Your posture automatically improves, your demeanor takes on a "Hey, I'm terrific" lilt and you feel stronger, more secure, smarter as well as prettier than when you first met your morning face in the mirror.

Does it sound complicated? It's not. As soon as you've put in a few practice sessions, your makeup should not take more than fifteen minutes to complete. Even my grandmother got it down pat after she had her makeup session for this book.

Makeup—Step by Step on Susan Phillips

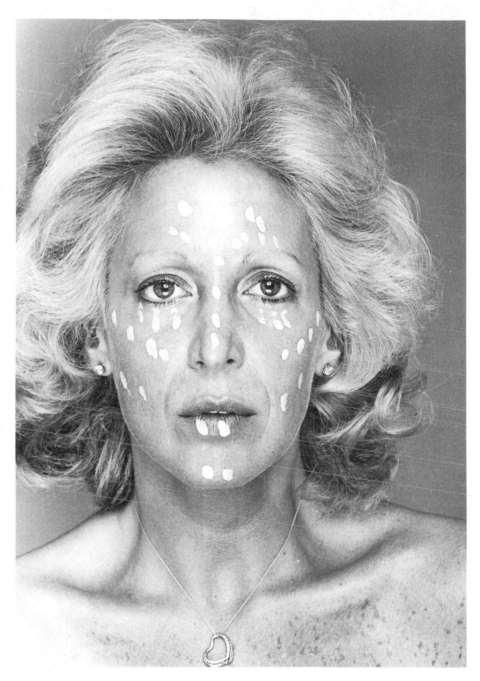

The makeup base has been spotted on,
soon to be blended smoothly.

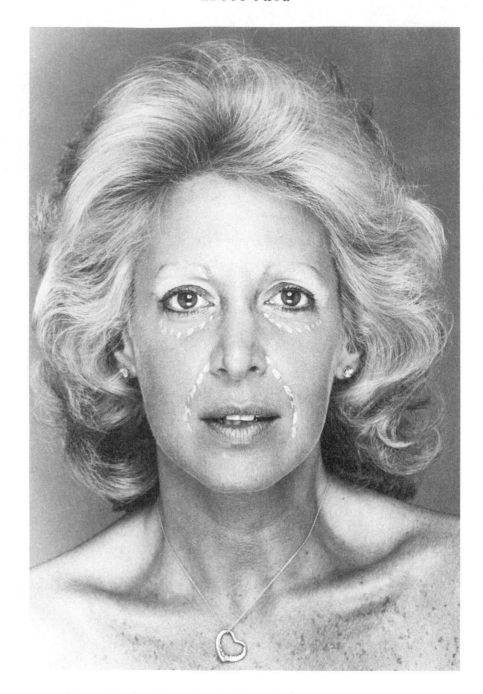

Concealer has been spotted on circles under the eyes
and on the lines that run from nose to mouth.
This will also be blended smoothly.

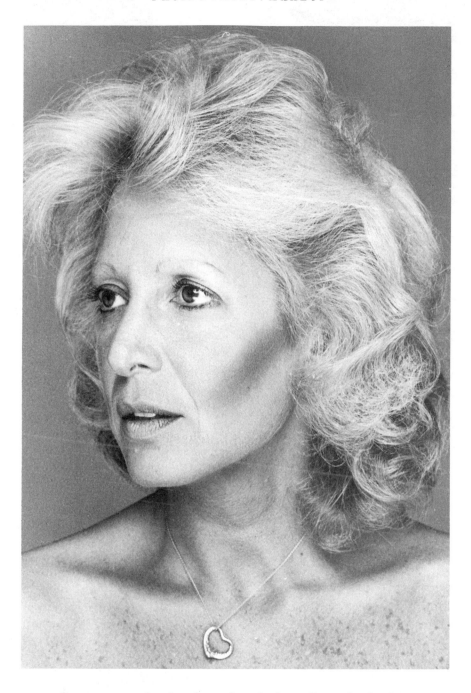

Contour powder has been brushed on Susan's cheeks
and forehead in a parentheses shape
that frames the eyes.

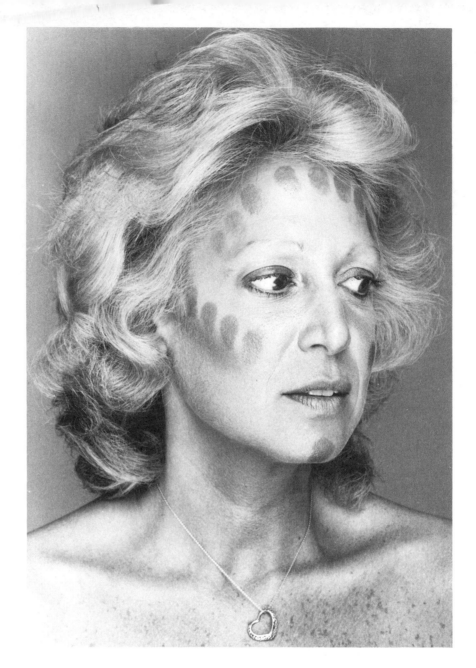

Cream rouge has been dotted on the cheeks and forehead following the line of the contour powder. A spot of rouge has been placed on the chin. It, too, will be blended softly so no distinct lines of makeup remain. Note the uneven brow-line which must be filled in and the slight puffiness over the eyes which gives a tired, droopy look.

The brow color, in a shade that matches the natural brow has been brushed in. The primary eye shadow color, an orchid powder to accentuate the iris color, has been brushed onto the lid. Under the brow burnished gold highlights and meets the orchid lid color, making the eyes look larger and wider. The third shadow, an emerald powder, was added in the outer corner to widen the eyes and create distance between them. The last shadow, a charcoal softly smudged in the corner, joins the nose bone and the brow and gives depth to the eyes. Marine green crayon has been used in the wet ledge, and soft charcoal crayon smudged under the lower lash-line and over the upper lash-line.

Susan's lips have been lined with a lip pencil and the line smudged into the lip to erase a harsh, coloring book outline. Plum rose lipstick and gloss complete the picture.

She has a lot of makeup on but Susan looks natural, pretty and sparkling. Her eyes are luminous, her face more beautifully shaped and tinted—she looks younger and happier. The older you get, the less makeup you need? Wrong.

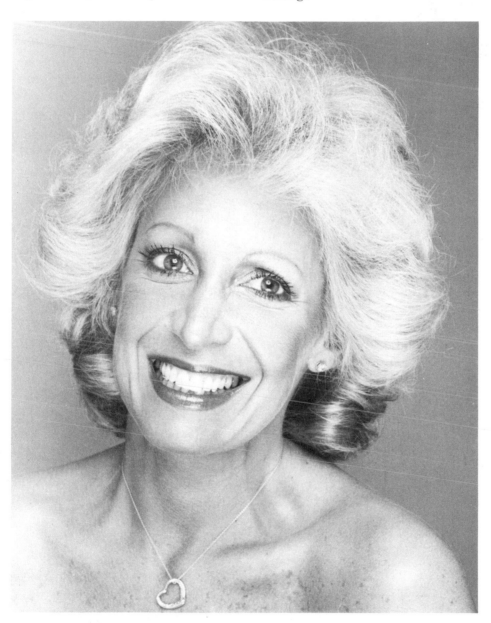

For a look at Susan in living color, see the color makeovers following page 112.

Tips and Tricks

First get the general makeup regimen down pat. Then, consider some of the specific tricks to subtly hone the art. What follows are tricks of the trade that every makeup artist worth his salt knows. They may look like magic but they're really sleight of hand; cosmetic surgery without a knife. They camouflage and make beauty where none existed before. Here's a cornucopia of makeup sorcery.

EYES

✳ To make the eyes appear larger, more slanted, *very slightly* extend out the smudged eyeliner under the *lower* lid to barely meet the eye shadow wafting out from the lid. The finest line of yellow *under* the darker, smudged eyeliner makes the eyes appear enormous.

✳ Only line *inside* of lower lid if your eyes are very large and wide-set. Lining inside the lash-lines can be dramatic but tends to make eyes look smaller. If your eye whites are not-so-white but yellowish and watery besides, and your eyes are reasonably large, line the inside lower rim of your eyes with a Nile-green or cobalt-blue pencil, which will make the whites look whiter by contrast.

✳ If you have a shaky hand and the eyeliner pencil always ends up a quarter of an inch away from your lash-line, try this technique. *Dot* on eye color as close to the lash-line as you can get: Then, with a Q-Tip, gently *connect* the dots in a smudgy, soft line. Be careful all dots are smudged uniformly together or your eyes will look like a connect-the-dots coloring book.

✳ You can highlight the roundness of the eyeball by putting a touch of gold or pearly shadow just in the center of the lid—*never* a white dot!

✳ Eyelining pencils can come in terrific colors, but still be useless because their consistency is not right for the effect you need. When a pencil is too soft, sometimes refrigerating it for an hour will harden it. If the point is too hard, just hold the tip between your fingers for a minute or so to let your body warmth soften it.

✳ If your eyes are shot through with tiny, red capillaries, stay *away* from violet, pink or purple eye shadows which will accentuate the pink murkiness.

BROWS

✳ You can lighten very dark brows by bleaching them. Buy and prepare a packaged facial-hair bleach and apply it to your brows for a minute and a half or two minutes—stay away from the eye with the bleach! Remove bleach with a cotton pad and carefully wash brows with soap and water to get *all* bleach off. This will mute the intense dark color but will not turn your brows white or blond (unless you leave the bleach on for longer than the prescribed two minutes).

✳ Brows are best plucked at night, before sleep to give the traumatized area a few hours to rest and reduce any puffiness. Always dab the brow area with alcohol after tweezing, and moisturize. If you apply makeup right after tweezing, there's a good chance that the newly created opening left by the tweezed hair can clog and create a pimple or infection. Alcohol tends to close and heal the pore where the offending hair existed.

❋ To correct a too-thin brow try brushing the brow hairs down and then, with a sharp pencil, feather in the missing "hairs." When you brush your brow back up with a soft toothbrush, your own real brow hairs will blend in nicely and cover the pencil additions.

❋ Just before the theater you notice an unruly eyebrow hair; you tweeze it and— disaster!—a swelling as big as the Ritz, not to mention the redness. Before you tweeze that hair, try a fast application of ice on the area, for about three minutes. That freezes the area, eliminates swelling and by constricting the pore almost pushes the hair out. What's more, a little freshener dabbed onto the plucked spot prevents redness and closes the newly vacated pore.

LASH TRICKS

❋ Vaseline makes them grow longer—I promise!

❋ When you curl your lashes, make sure you vary the pressure by vibrating the curler a bit as you hold for about ten counts. Release handles completely before you pull the curler away.

❋ How can you get the most uniform color on the mascara wand? Most people pull the wand in and out of the container which creates an imbalance of color on the wand and dries out the mascara by letting the air rush in and out. Simply pull out the wand very slightly and slowly rotate it within the container. This gets an equal, thick amount of blackness on the wand and preserves what's in the container.

❋ If you must wear false lashes, natural looking, *individual* lashes look best. Before removing any false lashes, dab on some baby oil to loosen the adhesive. What if you haven't the dexterity to handle individual false lashes? Here's a trick to make the whole band of lashes fit much better. Take the edge of a very blunt knife or the non-cutting edge of a closed manicure scissors; holding the band of the lashes between your fingers in one hand, with the other pull that blunt edge of the knife or scissors right along the eyelash band. This gives an even curve to the band (and the lashes) so it adheres smoothly and naturally to your own lash-line.

❋ Oil the rubber on your eyelash curler, as well as your lashes, for smooth, non-pull curling.

❋ Apply two coats of mascara (allowing each to dry in between) on *both* sides of the top and bottom lashes.

❋ If your eyelashes look clumpy, separate them by brushing them with a toothbrush or special eyelash comb or brush.

LIPS

❋ Slightly yellow teeth? Avoid yellow-based colors like gold or orangy-rust shades. Stick to roses, plums, soft reds which have a blue base and will counterbalance that yellowish cast of the teeth. Your lipstick texture should have a soft gloss to it rather than a matte finish which will focus the attention on the lips and not the teeth.

❋ Make sure you *blend* the burgundy pencil lip liner: An obviously outlined mouth looks unappealing and like a follow-the-lines drawing. Lip pencils, by the way, should be hard, not soft—the opposite of eyeliner crayons which should smudge easily.

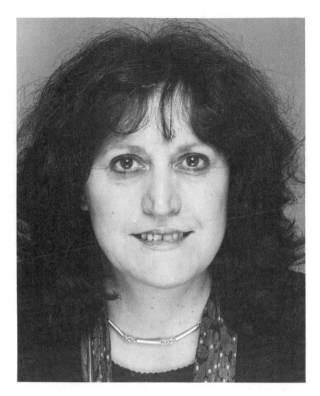
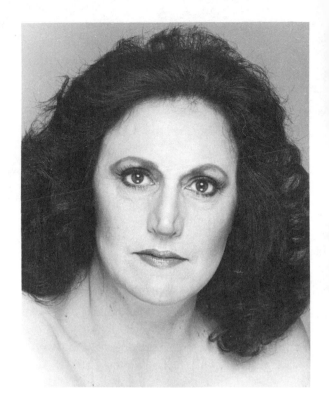

JUDY LOCK

* Puffiness of the jowl area can begin right by the cheek and not at the chinline: Make sure your burgundy lip liner draws an infinitesimal *lift* right at the lip corner instead of a downward line. That will draw attention *away* from the beginning sag of the jowls and make a sad-sack mouth into a positive, sensual mouth.

* Lips can take on a delightful pout if you put a golden (or any lighter-than-your-lipstick gloss) tone just in the center of the lower lip. Blend in well, of course.

* For a long face: avoid the valentine "bow" shape at the top lip.

* For a very heavy, squarish jawline: paint the heaviest intensity of color in the middle of the mouth, not at the sides.

* For a rounded face: paint lip liner on with more defined, sharper bow. Bottom lip should not be "pouty" and rounded: It should have a broader sweep.

* Never try to make both sides of your mouth *exactly* even.

* Do you have a too-thin lower lip? Check in a mirror to find your "delta"—the triangle-shaped shadow that's directly in the center—just below the lower lip. Draw your lip-line a *fraction* below the natural lip-line and then, softly, with a tiny brush, shadow in the delta with contour powder. Blend and gently dust with powder. When you put lipstick on, you'll note how much more seductively full your lower lip appears.

CHIN

* To hide a double chin, give a stronger jawline to a weak chin and do the best you can for chin-sag contour along and *just under* the sides of the jaw with your warm, earthy-ruddy contour powder and a good sable brush. It works miracles!

* Bring the eye up! Use more eye color, more eye-makeup generally, to take the attention away from the lower part of your face.

FACE

* Does your makeup often look runny—as if you've been out in the rain? You need to prepare your face better *before* makeup application and use your imagination to find the right tools for cleanup. For instance: If you use an oily eye-makeup remover, you better get it *all* off or your eye shadow will surely run and smudge.

* Does your base look shiny and does it disappear quickly? It's too *moist,* or you're applying too much moisturizer before the base.

* Does your face look *more* wrinkly and lined and caky after the base you've applied than before? Try using a liquid as opposed to a cream for less thick consistency. Also, use your fingers to blend—not a sponge which lays it on too thickly.

* Is the coverage uneven and cakey in patches? You must blend better. Try some more moisturizer in the evenings before bed to provide more lubrication.

* Your skin is still ultra-dry, no matter how good a moisturizer you use? Make sure your face is slightly damp before you apply the moisturizer, which is supposed to *seal in* water, *not* provide all the moisture.

* To camouflage scars and pitted areas, layering is the secret. If you dot on several layers of concealer, you will actually fill in the pitted area or the scar. Put the concealer *in* the indentation before you apply the makeup base. Powder. Put on the base. Put on more concealer. Powder. Put on more foundation. Blend carefully. Do this several times until the pitted area is built up to the level of the rest of the chin. Blend and powder *lightly* after each application. Layering is not just for clothes.

STEADYING

Often, the difference between a professional looking makeup and an amateurish job is a steady hand. If you have a shaky hand, make sure you are sitting and have a table on which to rest your elbow. Make good use of the pinky and fourth finger as you press them against your face when you outline eyes or do other such applications requiring steadiness. Outline eyes not by *stretching out* the eye from the outer corner and drawing from inner to outer corner, but by *holding* the eye steady with the opposite hand *at* the outer corner and drawing from outer corner to inner: It gives far greater control.

BLENDING

Most women spend half an hour on their eyes and five minutes on their makeup base. Wrong. If the base is not blended into the under-chin and neck, you look like you're wearing a mask. You can blend with your fingers, with a small, *dry* sponge or with your brush and some translucent powder.

STAINING

Okay, the makeup looks terrific—on your face. It doesn't look so great on your blouse. How do I remove makeup stains? Greasy, stubborn spots left by lipstick, blusher or foundation come off best with a strong, dry-cleaning solvent like K2r Spot-lifter. For powder, mascara and eye shadow spots, try Carbona Cleaning Fluid or Afta Cleaning Fluid. For emergency clean-ups when you don't have any solvent handy try this for washable fabrics: Scrub a stain with a toothbrush dipped in baking soda and water, let dry, then brush with clean toothbrush. Or—believe it or not—hairspray will remove many makeup stains.

Freebies

Not makeup freebies but wise words. I strongly suggest that you send away for the following free booklets which will educate you in the buying and using of cosmetics. Remember that cosmetics are chemicals and the intelligent cosmetic consumer should educate herself to their pros and cons.

Eye Products: Handle with Care; booklet no. FDA 73-5004 (How to buy, use and store eye-makeup)

Safe Use of Eye Cosmetics; booklet no. FDA 75-5003

All About Cosmetics; booklet no. FDA 74-5004

ORDER FROM: Food and Drug Administration
HFJ-10 Consumer Inquiries
15 B32 Parklawn Bldg.
5600 Fishers Lane
Rockville, MD 20857

Cosmetics; booklet no. 568 F (How to read labels; ingredients; hypoallergenic makeup)

ORDER FROM: Consumer Information Center
Pueblo, CO 81009

When ordering, write *Free* on the outside of the envelope.

THE BIGGEST MISTAKES: WHICH ONES DO YOU MAKE?

It's funny about makeup: even a person who has clarity and good sense in every area of her life sometimes cannot see herself objectively in the mirror. That's because we fall into traps of habit. Do something often enough and it feels and looks right, even if it's glaringly bad. There are a few makeup blunder-patterns which are almost classic, because so many women opt for them. Look closely and honestly at these descriptions: Do you recognize yourself here?

TIME WARP

Someone once said, "If you've always done it that way, it's probably wrong." That's very wise. At fourteen, you stole into your mother's bathroom vanity and dabbed on your first rouge and lipstick, feeling for all the world like Mata Hari. Miracle of miracles, instead of hitting you the pimply boy next door said you looked pretty, and that positive feedback has lasted you nicely for

twenty years. You haven't changed your technique or lipstick shade since. Or your white Courrèges boots. Others, in the same time warp, wear long blond pony tails, eyeliner wings, navy-blue lip liner and ooh-ooh spit curls pasted on their faces.

Makeup styles have changed along with other fashion trends and with liberation. Your face has changed. What was attractive twenty years ago is not attractive now. You *feel* the same, but you didn't have eye-overhang in high school when the blue eye shadow changed your life—Believe Me. So break out of your time warp. You know, in your heart of hearts, that no one else is wearing the beauty marks any more.

THE GROUCHO MARX BRIGADE

There's a certain group of women in the forty- to fifty-year-old age range who were brought up to believe that wearing makeup is sinful and cheapening. Powder has never touched their faces; instead of lipstick they bite their lips to bring up the color; and foundation is for scarlet women. There is one exception: Somehow they've been brainwashed to think that eyebrow pencil is forgivable and not really "makeup." So, they pencil in their brows with a thick, blackish line and let the rest of their faces stay pale—all you see is brow.

DOE-EYES OF DEATH

Absolutely my most loathed makeup error. When you draw out eyeliner to extend beyond the natural eye (and some women go wild doing this, extending the liner to the hairline), it looks cheap and most unflattering. A look that was popular in the '50s when Cleopatra was the current makeup model, the doe-eyes of death immediately label you as the rankest amateur in makeup application.

THE RICE CAKE LOOK

It comes from applying face powder which has color added to it, and it makes you look embalmed. Charles of the Ritz, among other makeup lines, will blend your powder "personally," supposedly matching it to your face color. You end up looking like a Kabuki dancer who has just smeared a rice cake over her nose.

SHIMMER AND SHINE

One of the most common mistakes is to misread *moisture*, when the directions call for moisturizing. Moisture is not oil. Moisture doesn't shine. Moisture is fine. Shine is not fine. If you're twelve and you have a fresh, scrubbed, shining look, everyone wants to hug you. If you're twenty-one and you're shining, no one wants to hug you lest he get the shine on his suit. I notice many cosmetic companies pushing shine on the eyes now—an absolute abomination. Disco dust on a forty-five-year-old merely puts glitter in a wrinkle, and that wrinkle wriggles and writhes with each blink of the eye.

RACCOON EYES

I see them every day and it's all I can do to stop myself from turning to a woman on the street and saying, "No, no, no!" When using concealer to hide the puffs and lines under the eyes, too many women smear it all over the puff instead of just dotting and blending in the line of demarcation under the eye. Whitening that puff highlights it, making it puffier than ever and giving you white, raccoon-like patches under your eyes. Somehow, the look became fashionable in the '60s when Jean Shrimpton, the model, and Twiggy, the bean, popularized it. It's awful; it dates you; it does nothing for lines or wrinkles but accentuate them.

INVISIBLE LIPS

Or: *Oh God, where's her mouth?* Only a twelve-year-old entering puberty should wear light pink or no lipstick. If you're over sixteen you should wear color on your lips, even if it's a soft blend of color and gloss. If you put Erace or Pan Stick or another concealer on your lips, you have no lips. Simple as that. Those circlet "virgin gold pins" go with the Invisible Lip look.

THE WINSTON CHURCHILL LOOK

Many women must believe that if you draw lip liner above the natural lip-line, and then color in not only the lips, but part of the skin above the mouth as well, no one will see your natural lip-line. It looks silly, coarse, un-pretty and very, very dated.

MASCARA CLUMPING

It's usually awful, and can be pretty only if you're very young and very skilled. Anyone else trying to get that "starlet look" by clumping her lashes with mascara instead of applying it evenly only gets stuck-together eyelashes.

CHEEKINESS

In the dictionary, cheekiness is defined as impudence, but I'm afraid I'm a bit more literal. One of the biggest makeup mistakes women make is putting bright colored blusher and rouge under the cheekbones, along the hairline, in a hundred other wrong places. If you do that, your face will not only look fatter, it will look floozier. If you see a line of rouge ending just before your hairline, it's wrong! Blend! Cheek color is supposed to make you look healthy; not feverish, which is often the result of too much color. If you've accidentally put on too much blusher or rouge don't try to wipe it off with a tissue, which will only streak it: remove it with a dry sponge, add a little foundation or translucent powder to cover and start all over.

THE PHONY-BALONEY TAN

You don't need the clue of a white neck and a bronzed face to give it away. Bronzers look fake when they're obvious. Solution? Mix a drop of bronzer into your regular foundation if you *must* have a tan-like look and be sure you blend it well into the top of your neck.

THE LINED-GLOSS LOOK

Carefully outlining your lips with bright color and then painting in with *just* lip gloss looks terrible. And that's all I want to say about *that*.

GYPSY MADNESS

There is *nothing* worse than a painted-on beauty mark. If you insist upon this artifice, please add hoop earrings and a tambourine to complete the look.

SLASHES, DOTS, AND DASHES

Finally, one of the worst and most common mistakes is not blending color into color. Wearing makeup is fine: It says that you're a woman who cares about her appearance. But if people can tell just what makeup you have on, that's a problem of blending. A slash of color on the cheek or a hard line of contour looks vulgar instead of pretty. Blend with your fingers, the best makeup tools you have, and then blend with translucent powder to soften even more. Never apply makeup and just leave it there.

*

Can't decide what mistakes you're making, or even if you're making mistakes at all? *Solution:* Put on your makeup as you always do. Have a friend take a close-up color photograph of you. Then, have the photograph enlarged. Study it carefully. Show it to someone whose makeup sense you admire for suggestions. You might learn more from one picture than from a year of looking in the mirror.

Nine Big Mistakes

EDA ROTH—producer, actress, and very good friend—was also a very good sport. She allowed me to illustrate, on her face, nine of the biggest mistakes a woman can make with makeup. Look at the face top right. What's terrible about it? This is what's terrible.

1. Base too dark. It should be a half-shade lighter than natural skin tone.
2. Shine is blinding. Where's the translucent powder?
3. Brows too heavy.
4. Eye shadow layered on with no thought of blending. Eyeliner too obvious.
5. Lipstick glopped on thickly; color too light.
6. Lip liner not blended into mouth.
7. Raccoon eyes; blend that concealer! (It's not even concealer; it's frosted Erace.)
8. Contour is a stripe; blusher is too heavy.
9. Face and neck are different colors.

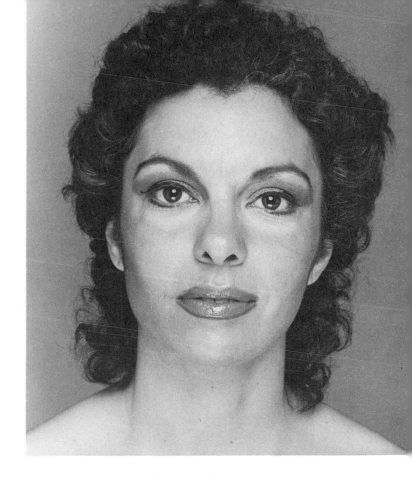

Here is the real Eda—softly made up, minus the mistakes!

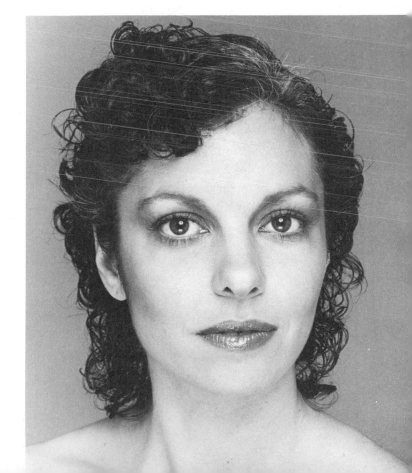

Let There Be Light

Don't even think of making up unless it's in the same light in which you'll be seen. If you expect to be outside in bright daylight most of the day, make up in the daylight. If you'll be inside in artificial light, you don't need the glaring truth of daylight. What's important is to see what others are seeing— no matter if you have trouble facing the new pimple. Light can alter the color of the makeup you apply and can dramatically change the effect.

If it's daylight where you'll spend your hours, find one of those mirrors that swing out on an extending arm and simply hook it over your window. Or, find one that stands on the floor and can be easily moved to the window. And don't be surprised if that great wine lipstick changes to an irridescent fuchsia when you see it in sunlight. Now, wouldn't you have died if you'd put it on under lamplight, unaware of its chameleon quality, and gone to the picnic looking like death warmed over? If you plan to be in daylight, you need a sheer foundation that won't look streaked. Concealers tend to look chalky in sunlight, so go easy here for outdoor wear. Because the sun intensifies colors, softer teals are more attractive than browns or greys which can look dirty in sunlight.

If you plan to spend the day in an office where fluorescent lighting is present, be aware that although it looks white, it gives a blue-green cast to all. That's great if you're wearing blues and greens in your eyecolor, but watch what it does to reds (turns them yellowish), yellows (turns them sickly sallow) and smoky greys and browns (turns them dirty). Generally, fluorescent light is hard and revealing, so you've got to check yourself out under them to see how to deal with your makeup. One area in your home should have some fluorescent lighting for you to make up under, especially if your office is lit with fluorescents. Lighter on the rouge and heavier on the blending blusher and powder is generally the rule. Makeup should be matte not shiny because the latter will even more strongly reflect fluorescents. If concealer in the sunlight is to be avoided because it reflects bright, natural sun, you'll want to wear it under artificial light because that intensifies under-eye shadows and bags and it does *not* intensify the concealing liquid. Blusher and rouge should have a touch of blue in them; light burgundy, for instance, has blue in it.

Incandescent lighting is much softer; it hides under-eye circles, provides warming glow and in general gives you more leeway to wear brighter color. Yellow tones ought to be avoided because artificial lighting of all sorts tends to give a yellowish tint to skin. Pinker tone in your foundation is called for. If your foundation doesn't come in the tone you're searching for, add a touch of color from a bottle of liquid rouge to your usual foundation. But by all means, look your prettiest when you're the boss, and that means makeup.

Dining by candlelight is, of course, the ideal light for young and old, because it does such wonderful things for your face. You can't apply makeup in candlelight (unless you're very weird), but you should be aware that although incandescent light casts wonderful shadows, those shadows *can* deepen any bags under your eyes. So be sure you go heavy on the concealer if you're toting those valises. Rich reds are fine for your lips and cheeks—much better than brownish earth tones which darken under candlelight and make a woman of thirty look fifty. Your eyes will look fabulous with the gem shades of emerald and amethyst.

So, when at all possible, make up in the light in which you'll be seen and understand what that particular light does to colors. Then you know what that new, Cary Grant-ish guy is seeing.

INVENT YOURSELF!

God and genes and shoddy luck may have put the wide nose and the thin lips there, but God doesn't mean you to live with them. Beauty is an illusion to be created by makeup when you weren't born with the violet eyes to die from. It's my belief that you can and should reinvent the way you look by using the tricks of the makeup trade, in much the same way that you can reinvent the way you buy goods and services by being an informed consumer.

The trick is not to hide the flaws. You can tell just how well *that* works by checking out each balding man who parts his hair near his ear, grows what's left to shoulder length, then flips those sparse hairs backward, and greases them down so they'll stay put in a futile attempt to conceal. Everyone seeing this silently says, "Jerk! Do you think *that's* attractive?"

Look at my picture on the back flap of this book. Unfortunately, I have the same hair problem as the "jerk" I've just described. I wish I had as much hair on my head as Brooke Shields has on her brows. But I don't. So I divert attention by playing up something else. I grow a beard. Your attention is drawn to my chin and not to a weak attempt to conceal. The same principle holds for makeup. The best way to minimize attention to a facial flaw is to play up something else, draw subtle lines and shadows that either direct attention elsewhere or mute attention to the actual problem. What follows are ways to deal with less than perfect faces.

Invent Your Eyes

Worlds can be conquered by eyes! And when it comes to eye makeup, the name of the game is individuality—perhaps more than with any other feature or facial area. I've said elsewhere in this book that our faces are not as unique as we think, and basically the same makeup techniques can be used for most of them, with the possible exception of the eyes. A woman with close-set eyes simply cannot apply shadow, mascara and eyeliner in the same places that a woman with wide-set eyes can.

Eyes that are not wonderfully sized or shaped by genes should be made more lovely by makeup carefully and individually applied to suit the specific problem.

CLOSE-SET EYES

Shade like mad out toward the temples, starting at the outer half of the eyelid and area under the brow. Of course, you'll softly blend to the inner corner of the eye with a lightened color so no sharp color delineation is obvious. Concentrate the deepest shades on the area going toward the hairline. Use your lash-liner on the outer two-thirds of the upper and lower lashes and also go heaviest with mascara on this outer two-thirds of the lashes.

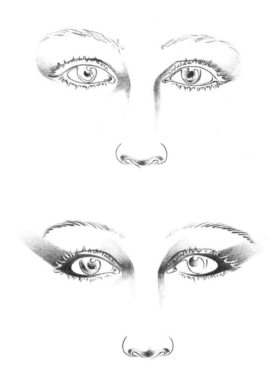

WIDE-SET EYES

Although these eyes are often lauded by makeup experts, sometimes they give the face a flat, vacuous expression. Jackie Onassis understands this, so she avoids heavy eye-makeup and always gives herself a strong, lushly colored mouth to detract from her very wide-set eyes. Shading heavily with shadow into the nose hollow is also helpful. (Wide-eyed women often have wide noses also, so check out Invent Your Nose.) When you line your lashes, do so inside the lower lid and apply mascara on the inner half of the upper lashes.

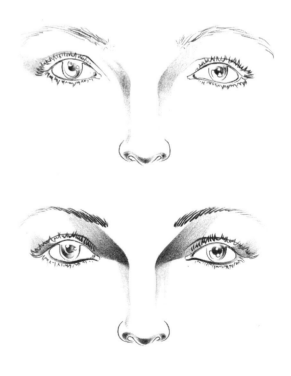

PROTRUDING EYES

If your eyes seem to be bulgy, your eye colors should be subdued earth tones. Soft colors on the outer two-thirds of the eye, extending up to the brow and well blended, will draw attention away from the eyeball that protrudes. Never use shining, disco colors (good advice for any shape eye). Choose a smoky, dark shade to recess the eyelid, and a lighter shade under the brow. Intensify color in the crease with a smoky grey or brown-black pencil.

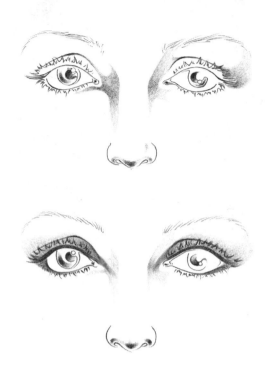

SMALL EYES

Here, you can use lighter, pastel shades on the lid, from the eyelid crease to the lashes. Then highlight, using a dark shade right in and slightly above the crease to create a wider eye. A light shade goes under the brow. Your eyeliner should be applied to the outer two-thirds of the lower and upper lash-line, and the mascara applied heavily from corner to corner.

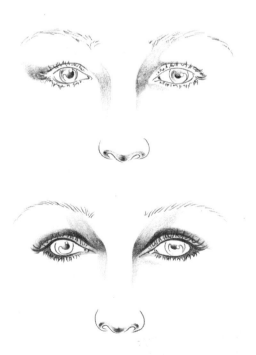

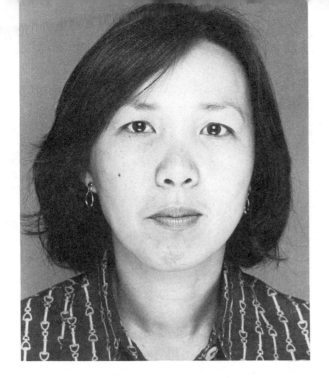
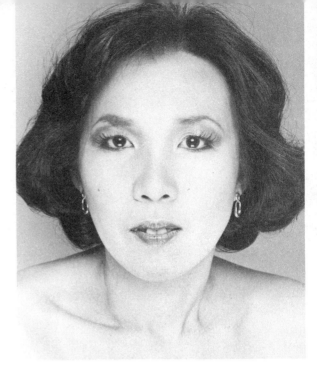

ORIENTAL EYES

Far from a flaw, oriental eyes can nevertheless be even more enhanced until they're spectacularly exquisite, if attention is paid to creating depth in the flat lids and dramatizing the wonderful almond shape. Observe law student GLORIA DiGENNARO's fine eyes, which were made delicately sloe-shaped by creating a "false lid." The actual lid is lightened with beige shadow and the eyelid crease darkened with a smudgy, smokey shadow. (Avoid a hard, dark shadow line on the lid, which will make you look like you have double eyelids.) The area close to the nose is also lightened, as is the under-brow area. Blended subtly in the outer areas (shadow number three) is a darker, duskier shadow. Remember to blend each of the four shadows into the others, each area intensifying and complementing the area next to it. Although I rarely use liquid eyeliner, it's wonderful on an oriental or narrow-lidded eye: apply it to the lash-line from inner to outer corner with the line widening slightly on the outer end of the top lashes. The effect is stunning. I shaded under Gloria's cheek-bones with contour to dig them out grace-fully and to bring attention to the lustrous eyes. Finally a rosy blusher and cream rouge give radiance to her skin, which has a ten-dency toward sallowness.

HOODED EYES

Otherwise known as eye-overhang, this is not necessarily a problem of aging. I've seen very young women with lids so heavy the eye seemed to be obscured. Correct this by applying your deepest color at the inner corner of the upper lid, extending it diagonally (as opposed to circularly) from the eye to the brow. Remember: darkness hides, lightness brings

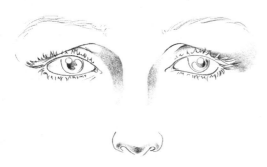
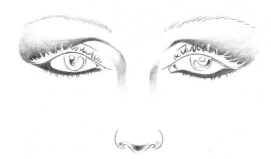

out, so use a warm brown shadow—not a pastel, ever! Your heaviest mascara will be applied to the upper, precurled lashes. It's very important, especially for you, to brush your brows upward, creating more of an arch and more room for shadowing under the brow to detract from the hooded area. So, the rule for eye-overhang is: darken the hoods to make them recede, play up and lighten above the eye and under the brow.

MARILYN COOPER, the popular actress who received a Tony award for Broadway's *Woman of the Year,* has this problem, along with millions of others. Soft taupe eye shadow on the ledge seems to make the overhang recede and lighter shadow under the

brow opens the eye up. Shadowing in a diagonal, for the third shadow, up to the brow further opens it and the fourth shadow in the corner of the eye gives depth. Smudged eyeliner under the lash-line extending *slightly* out beyond the lower lash-line works well. Brushing up Marilyn's low hanging brows gives her face more height and contouring around the eyes in a parentheses shape changes her long, droopy face shape to a wonderful oval.

No two eyes are precisely the same, so don't aim for precisely the same makeup application on each eye. Slight differences in shape, color and brow-line are natural looking.

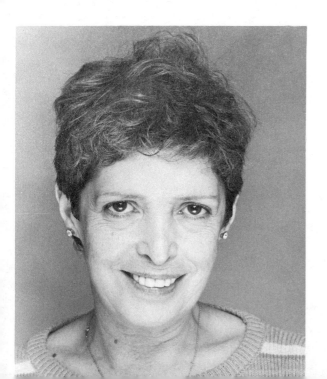
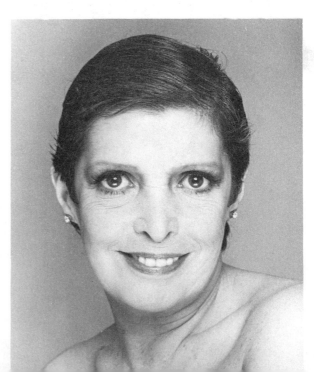

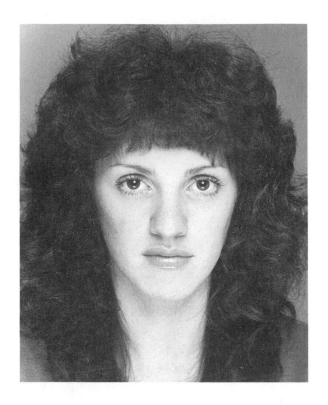

Invent Your Nose

"What's in a nose?" asked Cyrano. Plenty. Although it can't mirror the soul as the eyes are said to, or express a mood as the mouth does, the nose counts! As the center of your face, it serves as a focal point and reference for the other features. You really shouldn't be able to notice a nose too much, as opposed to the eyes and mouth which cry out to be noticed. Noses should just *be* there quietly, giving strength and dignity to a face.

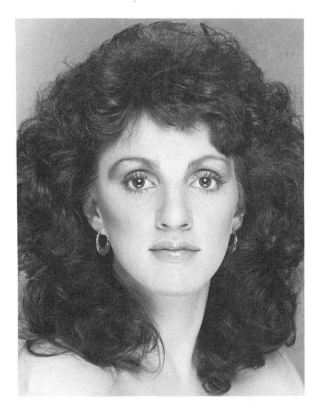

WIDE NOSES

Applying contour on each side of your nose can definitely narrow it, as shown in the photograph of Broadway's extraordinary star of *Evita*, TERRI KLAUSNER. People with wide-set eyes usually have wide noses and contouring the sides with a darker shade than the foundation you use gives it a more aquiline appearance. If you don't do it subtly, you will appear to have a dirty nose. Brush a mere suggestion of contour on the tip of the nose. Smooth and blend the dark shading until there's no strictly outlined area painted on the sides.

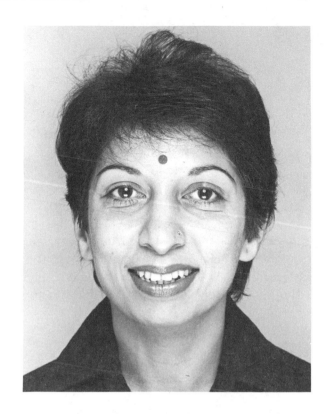

HOOKED OR LONG NOSES

Sometimes, the makeup illusion of taking off just a millimeter from the length of a nose works far better than surgery could. NILA GANDHI's nose was contoured right down its center and then the powder was blended well with my fingers. Translucent powder took away a ''stripe'' look. The merest touch of contour brushed on the top of the nose shortened it, as well. Concealer on Nila's dark eye-circles gave more room on the face for the nose, which also made it seem shorter and narrow.

TOO-SHORT NOSES

Believe it or not, they happen! Use a lighter shade of foundation, or a drop of concealer mixed in the foundation and apply down the center of the nose (lightness brings out, darkness hides) to give it more prominence.

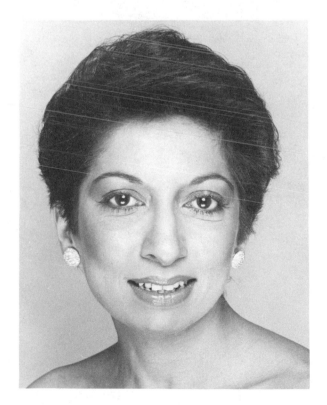

Invent Your Facial Bones

THE PILLSBURY
DOUGH BOY LOOK

He's cute but he's dish faced. There's not a bone in his face—no planes, depths or curves to give him facial character. This cute little guy has tushy cheeks. America's darling, Pia Zadora, would look like the Pillsbury Dough Boy if she didn't understand about contouring.

MARCIA LEWIS, Broadway's showstopper as Miss Hannagan in *Annie,* has a round face which deep-toned contour powder—brushed on under the cheekbone and out towards the temples—angled beautifully. Softer eyebrows and heavily mascaraed eyes gave further interest in her exuberant face.

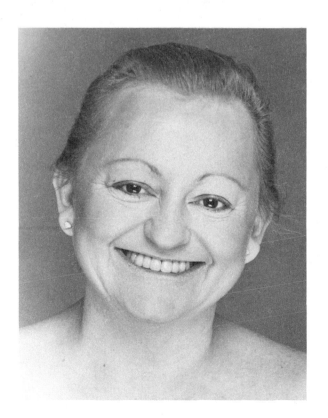

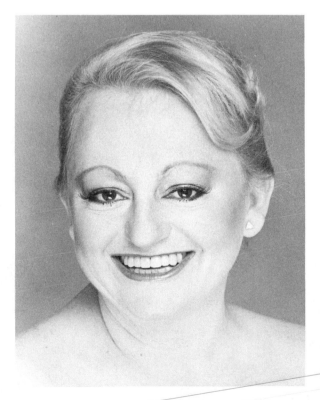

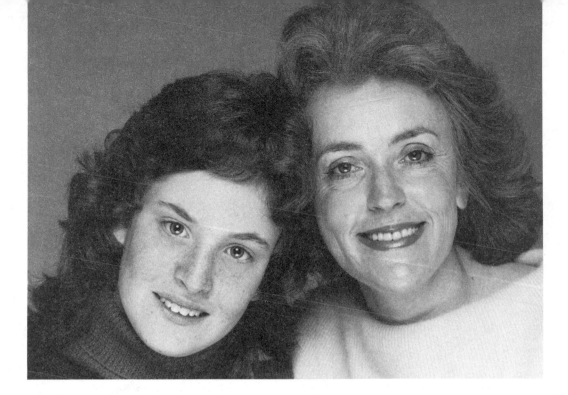

THE VIKING PRINCESS LOOK

Sometimes, one has to know when *not* to make up. If your bones are already prominent and wonderful, you don't need additional contour that will give you a skeletal or decidedly Viking look. If contour is applied at all, let it be in a semicircle under the cheekbones to widen the face, rather than dig out cheekbones that are already there. SHEILA and FRANCIE WEISLER, mother and daughter with the same narrow, beautiful, angular facial lines, are made up this way with a bit of soft peach blusher dabbed on the chin to soften it. Eyes and hair should be heavily played up to give facial symmetry. Francie's makeup, naturally, is much lighter than her mother's.

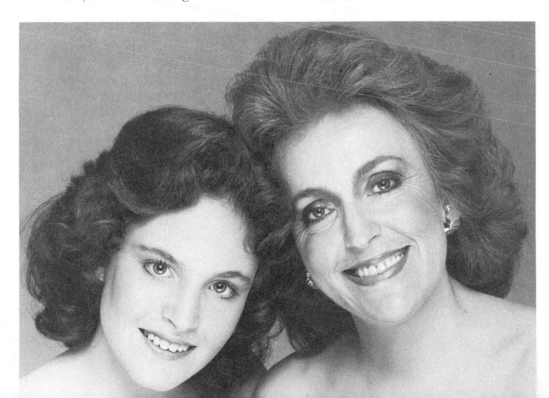

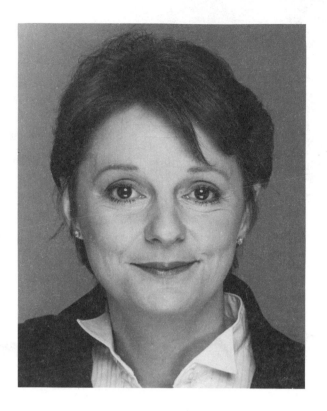

Invent a Chinline

CAROLE SHELLEY, Mrs. Kendall in the long-running play *The Elephant Man,* has a wonderful face that can be made even more wonderful with a more defined chinline—a sharpening of the facial contour. Many women, from age or genes, are plagued with jowls around the neck and chin. You can almost paint away a fleshy chinline if you do it properly. You can reduce two chins to a manageable one chin in the same way. Gently brush contouring powder right along your underjaw line, from ear to ear, using a wide sable brush. Then fill in the whole area with contour powder, painting out the loose or hanging jowls. For a double chin, brush a bit of the contour down the center of your chin, under your neck, and blend outward.

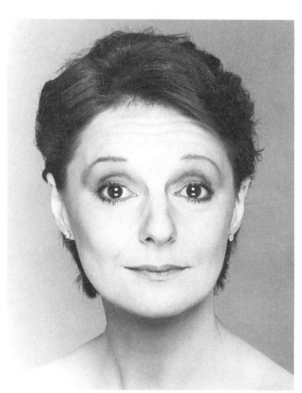

Invent Your Eyebrows

In makeup, the higher the arch of your brows, the more room there is under them to work with color, and that's what opens eyes up. I loathe bushy eyebrows, even if Brooke Shields has given them a certain popularity. It's a good idea to get them shaped professionally, at least once, just to give you a good line to work with. And make sure the makeup artist doesn't try to totally reshape your brows: It can't be done. He or she should simply follow the natural line and create the best possible arch, clean up the whole act by tweezing stragglers and create a pleasing (not screaming) frame for your eyes. Brows should never be drawn on in a continuous line. If you have bald spots in your brow, after brushing the brow up, feather in the skin with tiny strokes that look like hairs.

Don't try to make the brows exactly even, and don't be afraid to just cut with a scissors those few hairs that don't add much thickness but are simply too long. Here are some eyebrow tips.

* A brow should never start out thick and taper to a squiggle. It should be almost the same width all the way across, thinning out slightly and gradually in the outer half.
* Spray an old toothbrush with hairspray and use that to brush your brows up. They'll stay in place nicely.
* Always tweeze what grows between your eyes.
* If your brow stops abruptly before it reaches the outer edge of the eyes, extend it with little hair-like lines to frame the whole eye.
* Consider the color: the key words are soft and unobtrusive. Too-dark brows can be bleached professionally; if you try to do it yourself, be prepared for orange brows.

THE SIMPLEST GUIDE IN THE WORLD TO YOUR BEST COLORS

Never go by your hair or your eyes to determine the colors that will most flatter you. It's your skin that sends you a true color message. Although skin shades vary, there are three basic categories in Caucasian skin: Sallow or Pink–White, Ruddy (a flushed, reddish look or many broken capillaries—the outdoors look), and Olive–Mediterranean. Here are the best color bets for each of those categories.

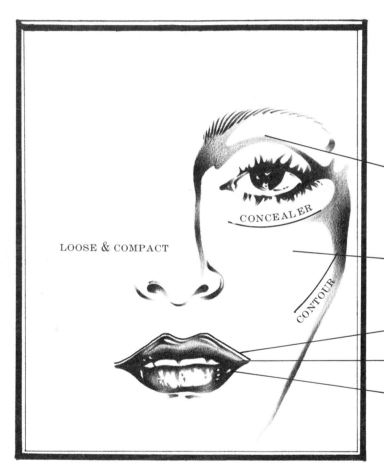

LOOSE & COMPACT

CONCEALER

CONTOUR

Sallow or Pink–White Skin

FOUNDATION: Avoid yellow tones; rose or peach tones are good

MASCARA: Black

EYE SHADOW: Blue-based colors—berry shades, mauve, violet, blues, orchid, purple, rose, pink
Try: gold, emerald

ROUGE AND BLUSHER: Pink lends rosy tones; if skin is more pale than sallow, peach will add a golden, warm tone

LIP LINER: Burgundy

LIP GLOSS: Clear

LIPSTICK: Almost any color looks good on you but make it a color in a flawless intensity; avoid muddy shades

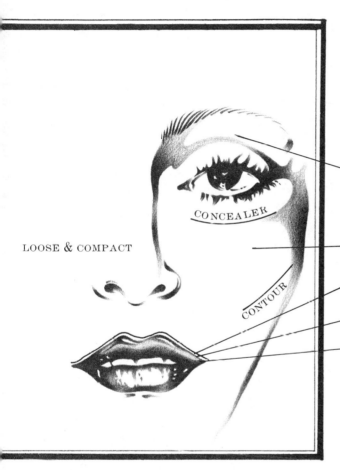

LOOSE & COMPACT

CONCEALER

CONTOUR

Ruddy Skin

FOUNDATION: Avoid reddish tones; go for peach tones

MASCARA: Black

EYE SHADOW: Earth shades—browns, greens, yellows, rust, copper
Try: mauve, magenta

ROUGE AND BLUSHER: Coral, amber

LIP LINER: Burgundy

LIP GLOSS: Bronzes

LIPSTICK: Burgundies, russets; avoid pink

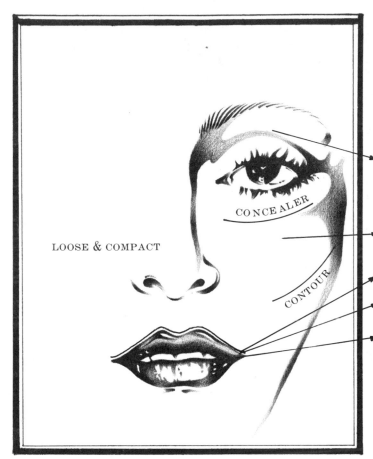

LOOSE & COMPACT

CONCEALER

CONTOUR

Olive–Mediterranean Skin

FOUNDATION : Light tan

MASCARA : Black

EYE SHADOW : Almost any shade ; pick up a tone of your skin or hair color or something you're wearing

ROUGE AND BLUSHER : Pure red and amber

LIP LINER : Burgundy

LIP GLOSS : Coral, cherry-red, clear

LIPSTICK : Earth or blue-based shades but best are pure reds and corals ; avoid bright pink and orange

GENERAL COLOR STRATEGIES

* Consider the colors that look best on you in clothing; they are often good makeup colors for you.
* Foundations should pick up a glint of your skin tone but be a half-shade lighter than your natural color.
* Color for makeup should not reflect the changing nature of the times, but only what looks good on you. For example: at the end of the '70s we saw a "new wave" mentality in color. Women tended to wear either no makeup or harshly aggressive colors. Flat, opaque reds and purples vied with sharply angled contour and haircuts. But, women who have discovered that they can be movers and shakers and still look feminine have dropped the trendy looks and adopted gauzy, translucent finishes, rosy hues, gentle angles—a sensual, womanly look.
* Lip color should be in balance with your eyes and the rest of your face. That's why the trend for Erace on the lips or no lipstick at all looked ghastly—it upset a proportional balance.
* Stay away from frosted colors unless you're very young: You can get a crepey-looking eyelid in five minutes from a frosted shade.
* Avoid glaringly bright colors: The prettiest shades are deeper, more muted.

Eye Shadow Color Combos

Generally, I loathe no-appeal charts and blanket statements. When I say that copper is a good eyelid color for a ruddy complexion, how can I know *how* ruddy your particular brand of ruddy is? How can you know *how* intense a brown, gold or shiny my brand of copper is? What follows, then, is a chart with some broad generalizations. You must be flexible and experiment with these color suggestions, which in my experience often look fine with the complexion types they're matched with here. Until you're sitting in my chair, though, I cannot be absolutely sure of the variations in your coloring, nor can you be absolutely certain what's in my mind when I speak of color. So, be adventuresome with these possible four-shadow combinations. Dare to be different!

Remember: *shadow one* goes under the brow; *shadow two* goes on the lid; *shadow three* goes on the outer corner of the upper part of the eye; *shadow four* softly joins the nose-bridge with the eyebrow.

SALLOW OR PINK–WHITE COMPLEXION

Shadow	*Combo 1*	*Combo 2*
1	Rose	Gold
2	Orchid	Pewter
3	Denim Blue	Lavender
4	Smoke Grey	Emerald

RUDDY COMPLEXION

Shadow	*Combo 1*	*Combo 2*
1	Peach	Mauve
2	Celery	Magenta
3	Copper	Teal
4	Toast	Brown

OLIVE–MEDITERRANEAN COMPLEXION

Shadow	*Combo 1*	*Combo 2*
1	Beige	Peach
2	Rose	Brown
3	Taupe	Smoke
4	Bronze	Mauve

THE VERSATILITY OF MAKEUP

The wonder of makeup is that, chameleon-like, it can change color and appearance. It lets you display your moods. Whatever your needs, makeup communicates the message just as powerfully as the tone of your voice or your clothing.

Suppose, for instance, you're going for a job interview, or, you are the boss conducting an interview and you want to make . . .

A VERY SERIOUS IMPRESSION

First of all, *Pull It Together.* Present a unified picture. Coordinate your makeup with your clothes. A tailored suit, for instance, does *not* call for eyeliner that circles your eyes entirely: that gives a wide-eyed, ingenue, little-girl look. A better technique is to line from the middle of the lash-line outward on both top and bottom lashes, which opens the eye more assertively, more chic-ly.

Colors: Pastels are definitely out. Sky blue, pink, gold or plum say fun and games not big bucks, big decisions. Lipsticks should be sienna, burgundy, soft coral—not cherry-red or fuchsia. Use smokes and taupes on the lids instead of brighter colors.

Eye shadows: Limit them to two or three. Eliminate the outer shadow that flares to the brow and maybe even the fourth shadow that connects the brow to the nose-bone. Keep them simple, soft, subtle. Eyeliners should always be smudged: Liquid liner is out.

Brows: Absolutely meticulous. Nothing says sloppy and disorganized faster than sloppy, unkempt brows. If yours are very pale, darken them: Pale eyebrows give a weak look; a washed-out demeanor lacking authority.

Overall facial appearance: Definitely matte. Oily shine says care less; matte says finished and efficient. Go light on the lip gloss. You want to have a clear, frank gaze: Nothing does it better than a soft, green liner in the wet ledge of the eye which dramatizes the whites of the eye and the steadiness of your gaze.

Carefully evaluate the whole look in the mirror: If anything on your face screams *sexy* or *exotic,* start all over. Above all, don't listen to the bores who say that makeup doesn't give an earnest, imposing impression. The respect you earn has to do with your talent *and* with the vibes you give off, and those vibes can be greatly enhanced when you look wonderful. You ought to look as good as you possibly can in your upward mobility climb. Looking dowdy or plain never won medals for anyone.

Suppose you're meeting The New, Wonderful Person at the tennis court, or, you're going out to lunch with your friend and you want to give . . .

A CASUAL, BREEZY, NATURAL IMPRESSION

First of all, *Think Glow not Glamour.*

Colors: Make them rich and light, not extreme. Tender mauve, pinks, denim, khaki, moss greens, peach and grey go on lids. Go heaviest on eye color, not contour or rouge. Blushers and rouges should be in warm peaches and pinks—it's the most natural: No one ever blushes in burgundy.

Eyes: Make your lashes a veritable thick fringe! A marine green or blue eyeliner makes them glow with spirit and life.

Complexion: Go with it! If it's sallow, use the yellow tones in the skin on your eyes. If you're very freckled, don't try to camouflage with heavy foundation—let them pertly accentuate your naturalness. The important thing is to even out the skin tone and that means, especially if your makeup is water or aloe based, to put it on quickly because it dries fast. Blend softly all with light powder dustings. If you have excellent skin tone or a terrific tan, you might consider a light, airy gel-type base.

Lips: Honest, bright colors are nicest. Clear reds, true cinnamon, soft pinks—depending on what you're wearing, applied *with* lip gloss for a luscious look. No-color lips are out: That doesn't spell natural—only boring. A colored lip gloss alone will do.

Suppose you want to give . . .

A SEDUCTIVE, GLAMOROUS, MYSTERIOUS, NIGHTTIME IMPRESSION

First of all, *Think Bones.* Nothing demonstrates the versatility of makeup more than contour powder. Use it to dig out your cheekbones or to recess your square chinbone or jawbone. You're not after a rounded, soft look or a jutting-out look, but an exotic, structured facial plane that's in balance.

Colors: Can be intense. Orchid-y, plum-y

eyes, for instance, are dynamite—purple eyes are grotesque. Pale glossy lips can have great drama and you can create a sexy dimple in the lower lip by shading the very center with a drop more gloss than the rest of the mouth (not Vaseline-gloppy—just glistening).

Eyes: Romantic, sexy, come-hither eyes can be created by extending the eyeliner on the *lower* lash-line very slightly out to meet the third eye shadow. The thinnest line of yellow, under a darker eye pencil line, makes your eyes glow with drama.

Disco dust and glitter stuff: Don't. Never confuse evening glamour with cheap, tawdry shine. Things that go sparkle in the night, like sequins or gold flakes, belong on go-go dancers not faces of sophistication.

Mouth: Wonderfully outlined, please, so your lipstick sensationally defines your mouth. A nebulous mouth erases a look of mystery and exotica.

No matter what impression you make with makeup, you want to keep it consistent. That means that the look you choose should persevere through several, even many, hours. Despite what the salesclerks at cosmetic counters say, makeup put on at 8 A.M. simply doesn't last until 10 P.M. You surely need to be familiar with the touch-up.

The Touch-Up Freshener

Sometimes you simply don't have the time to wash your face and start from scratch. You've got to touch up, intensify, replenish. Here are some tips on how to do it most efficiently.

* Biggest *must* is a compact of pressed translucent powder (as opposed to the box of loose powder you use in the morning). A few dabs of the powder obliterate shine and give a fresher look.

* A portable blusher with a small brush should always be in your makeup tote. There's nothing like blusher to wake up a tired makeup.

* You do *not* have to remove your lipstick for a touch-up. Just reoutline your lips and add a color and gloss combination.

* Never powder your lips, despite what you've read about that giving greater staying power. (Powder right *on* the mouth will dry it out faster than the Sahara.) If you want your lipcolor to last longer: put some lipstick on, lightly blot, *then* dust lightly with translucent powder, add your lipstick and gloss.

* Carry a tube of Vaseline. A bit added over mascara that's already on gives new shine and life to your lashes. You don't even need a mirror to do it.

* If you often go from office to nighttime activity, a good built-in touch-up device is to have your eyelashes dyed. It costs about twenty dollars, lasts six weeks and gives a lusher eyelash look—even when the mascara has worn off. Particularly useful to blonds with very fair lashes!

* It's always essential to carry a couple of Q-Tips in your makeup tote, for fixing smudged eyeliner.

* Finally, a word of praise for aloe-based foundations. They last. Even if you normally prefer something else, if you plan to be on the go from morning to late night, do use such a base for these times. You never have to worry about touching up such a foundation.

Molly Sharp

The incredible versatility of makeup is best seen by taking a look at Molly Sharp, a southern belle from Natchez, Mississippi, and how she changes her facial appearance as she moves through her life. "Makeup lifts my courage," says Molly. "It lets me be different people."

CASUAL CHIC

Going to market, playing a set of tennis, just "hanging out" call for a pretty speedy, splash-and-dash makeup for Molly. She puts on a layer of moisturizer as she always does whenever she wears even a very sparse makeup, because it acts as a protective barrier between her pores and the color. Today, she'll just spot on a porcelain base in strategic spots and blend it well. She curls her lashes, dusts a little gold shadow on her eyelids, a mauve shadow under her brows and puts on a light coat of mascara. A brush-on of apricot blusher and some pink-gold gloss and she's on her way out the door. It has taken three minutes.

OFFICE CHIC

Molly pulls back her hair for a more conservative look, applies moisturizer and a full face of porcelain base for an overall look of more sophistication. Her eye shadows are in a warmer family today, with peach under the eye, burgundy on the lid, khaki in the outer corners to open her eye and a golden smoke in the inner corner, joining her brow. She blends all, meticulously of course, puts on some amber rouge, the golden apricot blusher and a soft sienna lipstick. She grabs her briefcase, hails a cab, looks at her watch. It has taken eight minutes.

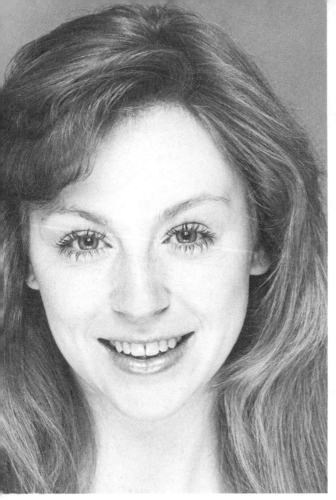

Casual Chic

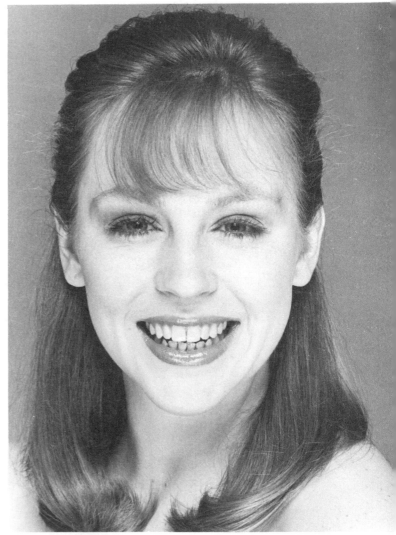

Office Chic

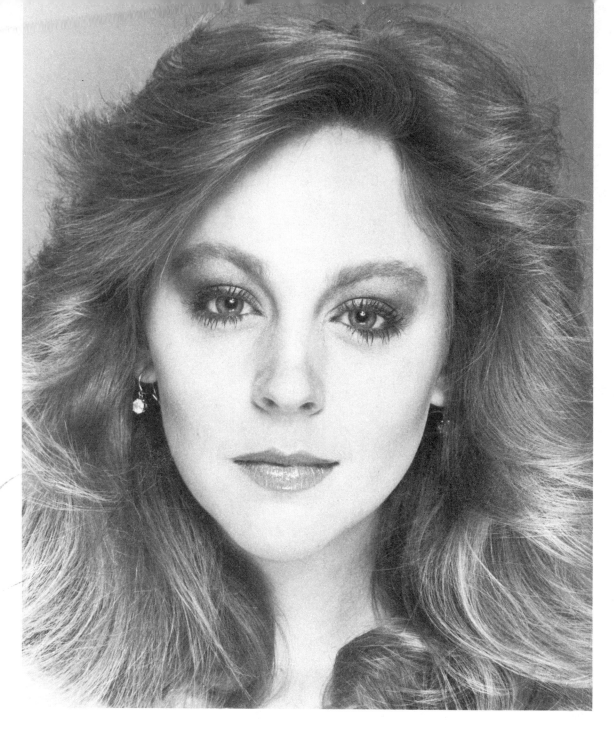

EVENING CHIC

All stops pulled out! Molly prepares for glamour and a smoldering look. The same porcelain base (her basic coloring doesn't change), but that's all that's the same. Contour sculpts out dramatic bones, and rouge and blusher are applied with a bit more inten-sity since the artificial evening light will soften everything. Lashes are curled in readi-ness for the two coats of mascara (on each side of her lashes). Brows are brushed up and filled in with brow powder. Eye shadows are now more romantic, more fanciful. Celery un-der the brow, rose on the lid, brown velvet in the outer corners and burgundy towards the nose give drama. A marine crayon in the wet ledge on the lower lash-line and smudged charcoal over the top lash-line and under the bottom line create softness and ethereal beauty. The lips are clearly defined and fuchsia lipstick blended with gloss makes her mouth irresistible. Naturally, her hair is brushed out in a wilder, more wanton look and—watch out world—here comes Molly! It has taken twenty-one minutes (including cleaning up).

The "Natural" Beauties

The truth behind "natural" is that it's very cultivated. Contrived. Worked at. That beauty with the Rebecca-of-Sunnybrook-Farm complexion has spent, no doubt, forty minutes in front of her makeup collection working at looking natural. Cheryl Tiegs, Christie Brinkley—those California girls, those natural girls—wear more makeup than you'd dream possible on such clear and shining faces. Natural is out . . . gorgeous is in. Makeup makes a plain face pretty, a pretty face magnificent and a "natural" face irresistible. Makeup gives you a confident, punchy, dynamite look. No makeup gives you the blahs.

Depending on natural beauty is silly. Maybe two people in the history of the world were natural beauties. The hype of the '70s—natural—was dishonest. The natural look depended on makeup, *just about always*. It was unfair and cruel to try to convince the American woman that all those models she saw running on the beach were natural beauties, when each came loaded with a ten-pound makeup case for the photography session. Learn how to put on makeup. Learn the secrets of skin care. Then you, too, can be a "natural" beauty.

4*

The Makeovers

IN MOST BEAUTY BOOKS, the reader is treated to stark *before* shots of absolutely clean-faced women and then, for huge contrast, to startling *after* shots showing the makeup artist's skill. While that may be dramatic, it's not realistic or honest. Most women know a great deal about makeup before they come for a professional lesson, and the trick is to show them what they're doing wrong and how to improve on what they're doing right, instead of assuming they're starting with zero talent. Therefore, the *before* pictures in this book were taken as my clients entered the studio with their daytime makeup applied. The *after* shots show what can be accomplished with good technique.

Naturally, it's always balance I strive for: the look of the *whole* face with each feature enhanced. Because each face presents many challenges, it's difficult to categorize makeovers into sections that illustrate makeup for one specific feature. However, it's been my experience that each woman usually has one feature, one area of her face that generally gives her difficulty when she does her own makeup.

The makeovers in this book, therefore, are grouped according to those areas, and although one must always consider the entire face, I hope the reader's attention will first be drawn to the way the "problem" has been corrected.

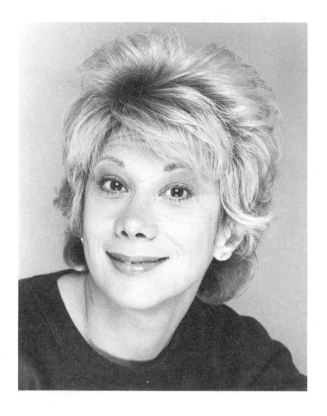

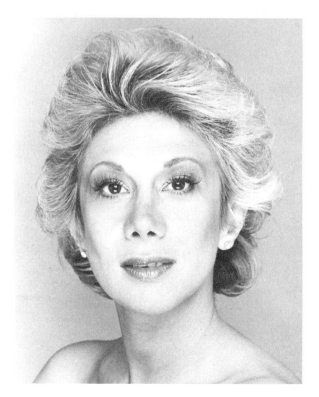

THE EYES

Perhaps no other feature can be so wonderfully enhanced as eyes. They're really *not* the windows to the soul, as legend has it, because even if you have a perfectly ordinary or an exceptionally sinister soul, your eyes can look angelic, luminescent, magnificent.

Marilyn Michaels

The popular television and club comedienne is probably best recognized from her Diet 7-Up commercial with Rich Little. Close-set eyes needed heavier shading in the outer corners to "pull" those eyes away from her nose and make them seem wider set. White concealer under the eye, deep purple in the outer corners to play up the natural almond shape, pink under her brow and pure gold on the lid ("Yellow?? You're putting *yellow* on my eyes??") made them spectacularly Egyptian without that black Cleopatra line that's so dated. A line of forest green starting at the center under the lower lash-line and playing out slightly beyond the eye, works far more magic than ringing the whole eye with green would. And, because crumbling mascara is one of Marilyn's biggest problems, the mascara was applied in a horizontal direction while holding the mascara wand vertically: That gives greater staying power as it lengthens and thickens.

CHEEKBONES—OR LACK OF THEM

"Dem bones, dem bones, dem—dry bones . . ." They're the secret of every elegant, sensual face, and if you weren't born with them, you can sculpt them out of the soft roundness you *were* born with.

Sherry Fritsch

At thirty-six, Sherry didn't look much older than her little girl and she thought it was about time to color herself with a little more sophistication. Shading under those fat, round cheeks brought her cheekbones into play and sultry beauty was born. Eye shadows matched the angle of the contouring, accentuated by a soft smudgy crayon under the lower lash-line, and angled out on the same slant—and sloe eyes were created.

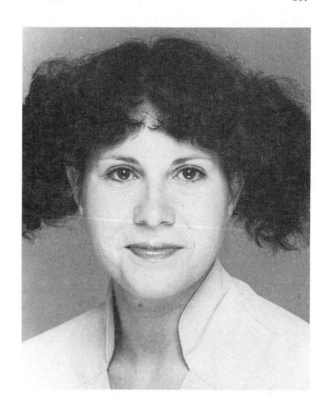

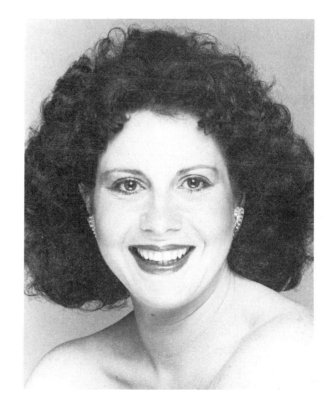

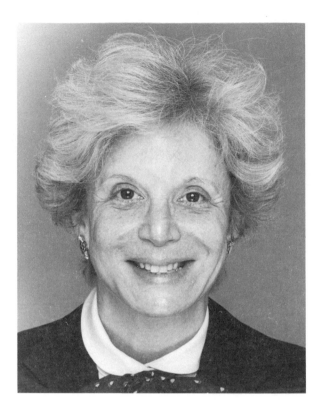 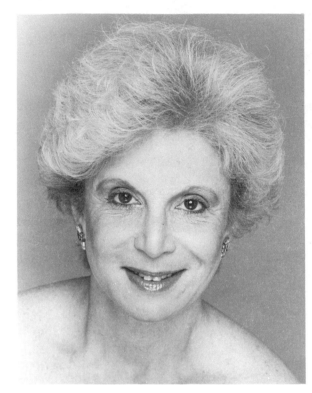

Sally Jessy Raphael

She's America's coast to coast radio advice columnist and she has "tushy cheeks" which are chipmunk-like pouches that hide any semblance of high cheekbones. I contoured in an inverted *V* with the point towards the hairline, one arm of the *V* going on a slant under the cheekbone and the other arm slanted halfway up the forehead. This had the effect of not only narrowing the cheek fullness but also the wide forehead. Titian rouge, an earthy coral color, followed the line of contour powder right *on* the cheekbone and golden apricot blusher, buffed quite vigorously on the contour and rouge, set both— to last all day and all night.

THE NOSE

No one should really notice your nose. It should just provide a pleasant but inconspicuous hub around which the more exciting features circle. But sometimes, a too long, wide, sharp or short nose demands center stage—and then, the magic of makeup should take over.

Darcy Pfifer

The all-American, girl-next-door star of Broadway's *Sophisticated Ladies*, Darcy has a sharp nose that dominates her face as her wonderful blue eyes and generous mouth go unnoticed. Contour powder on either side of the nose and on the tip brought it back into proportion and a well outlined mouth transformed her grin into a stunning smile.

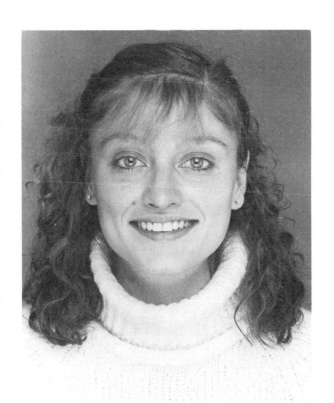

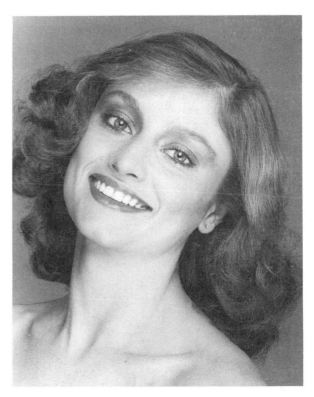

THE MOUTH

Lips are the face's most sensual aspect. They should be glistening not oily. Defined not nebulous. Inviting not scowling.

Stefanie Turnbull

She's my sister, and she came to my studio to be made up for her wedding day. When her eye makeup was completed, her mouth seemed lost with an upper lip-line that needed a clear definition. Outlining first with a lip pencil, I gave her a slightly fuller upper lip with a definite shape and filled in her mouth with a sunset coral color mixed with gloss. To complement the now fuller mouth, I powdered the inner corner of the eye with brown velvet shadow and joined that to the brow: This made the eyes seem wider apart and in proper alignment with her mouth.

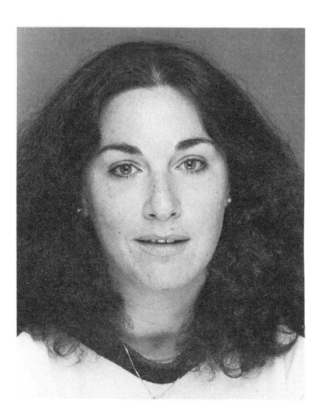

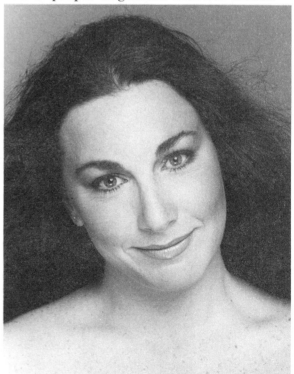

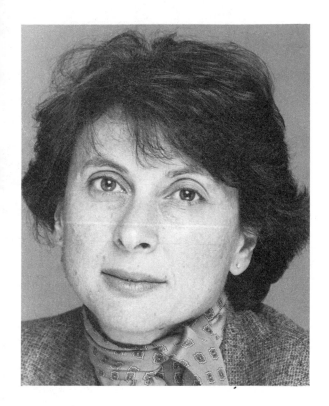

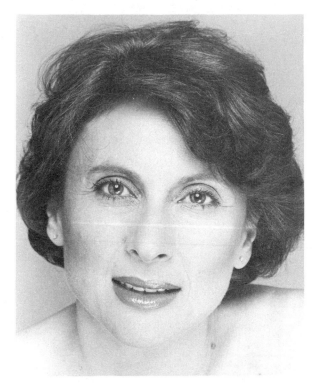

CHINS AND JAWLINES

Sometimes, the slightest muting of a too strong jaw or the most infinitesimal rounding of a pointed chin makes the difference between pretty and beautiful.

Allison Elliott

A shaker and mover in the book publishing business, Allison has a too-square jaw that was detracting from a wonderful smile and deeply expressive eyes. Contour powder on the jawline cut the bluntness and a well blended dab of rouge on the chin lengthened the chinline. "Parentheses" contouring under the cheekbone and up onto the temporal area framed the velvet eyes and brought attention there and away from the jaw.

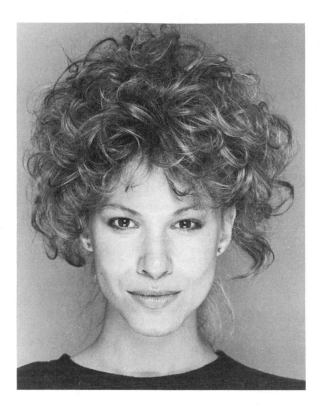 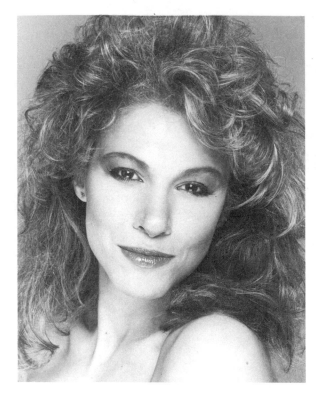

Debra Greenfield

An actress–photographer, charmer Debra has a long thin face, pointed chin and slightly narrowed eyes. The face shape was wonderfully enhanced with contour along the jawline to soften and with blusher right on the chin to round. Her cheekbones, already so dynamic, needed no help with contour at all—a case of more would be less. Eye makeup, heavier on the outer corners, pulled the eyes wider apart and that third shadow, joining the nose-bridge with the brow, gave instant depth and focus to the eyes. A vivid shade of lipstick on carefully outlined lips changed Debra from cute to seductive.

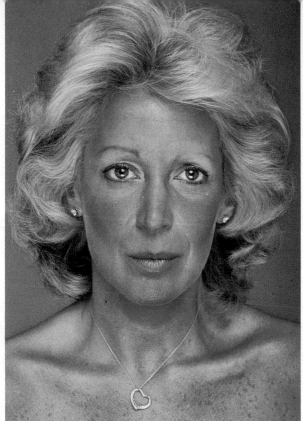

Before

Susan Phillips

(See page 72 for eye-makeup details.)

During

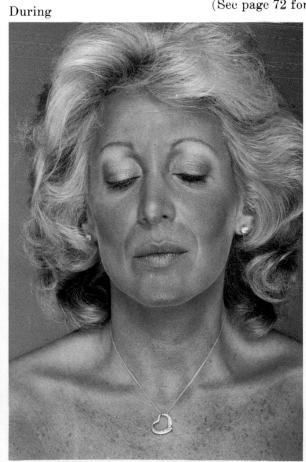

After

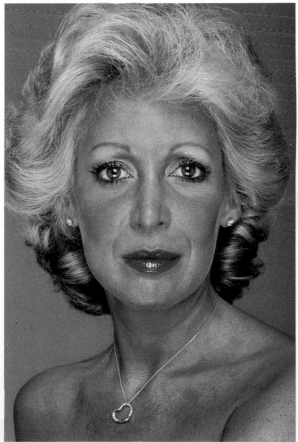

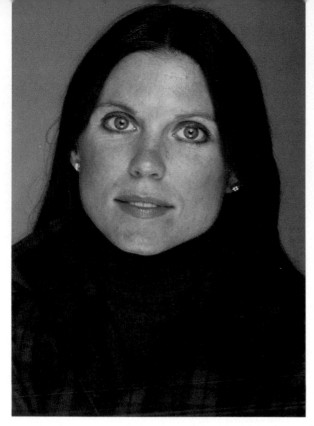

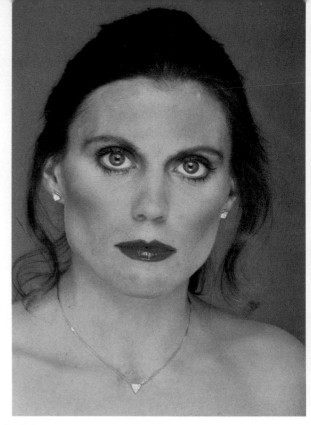

Ann Reinking
A pretty face can be an exquisite face. (See page 113.)

Elizabeth Hubbard
Makeup makes her "disappearing" tendencies disappear. (See page 113.)

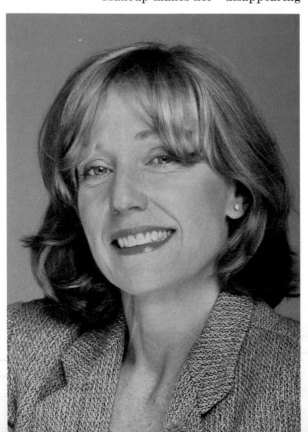

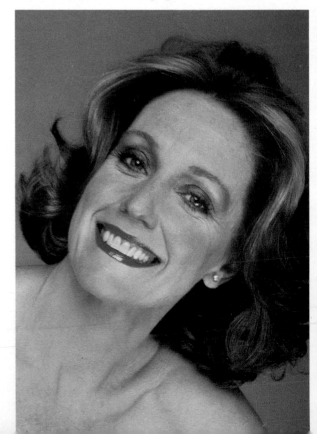

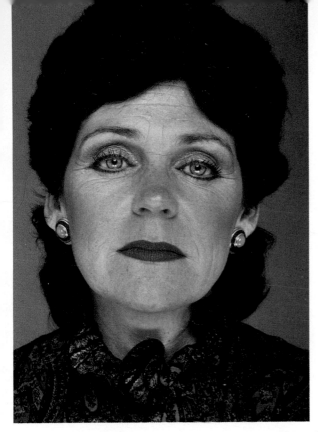
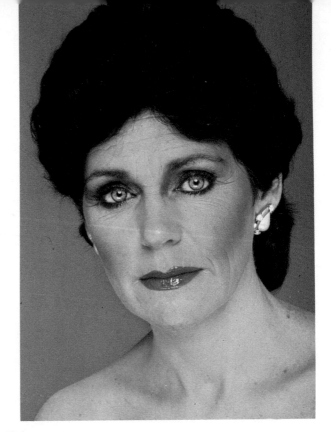

Carol Lipson

Makeup "overkill" transformed to makeup glamour and softness. (See page 113.)

Lizbeth Mackay

Transparent skin made wonderful. (See page 114.)

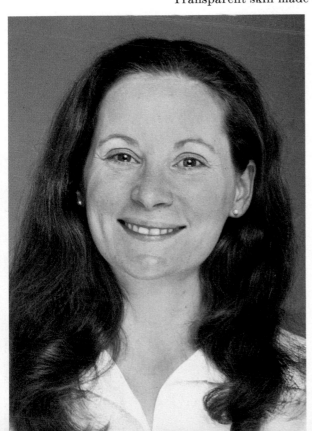
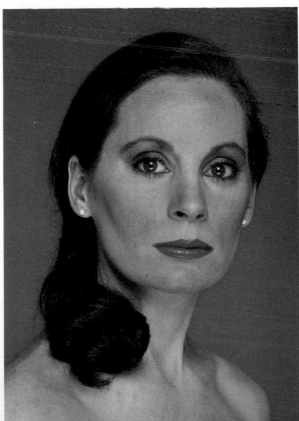

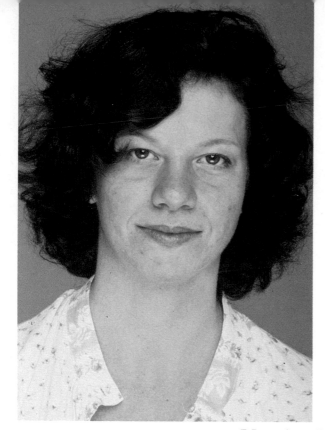
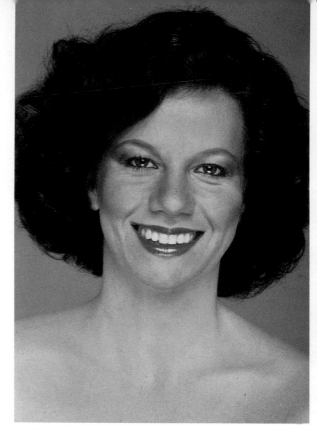

Martine Van Hamel

For drama and excitement, angles can be dug out of fleshiness. (See page 114.)

Dominique Singer

Sallowness and a washed out look are not irrevocable: color, properly applied, is sensational!
(See page 114.)

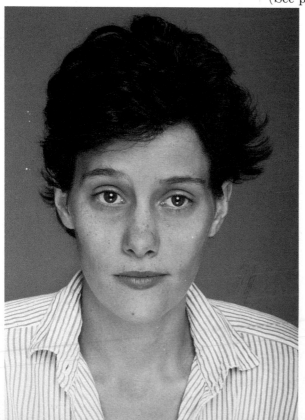
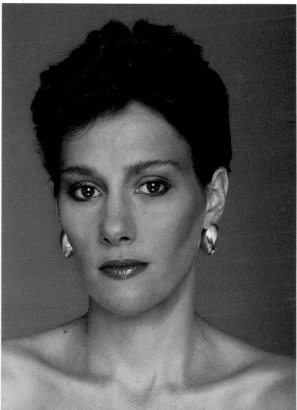

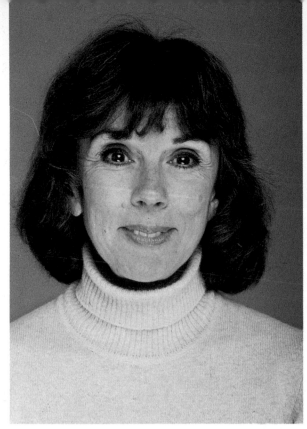
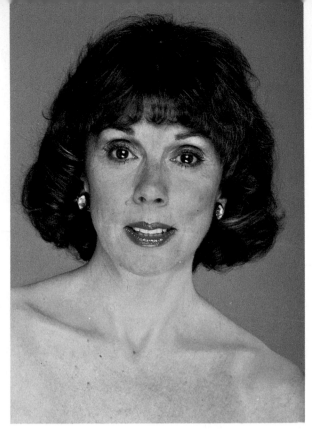

Phyllis Newman

"Always, always those dark circles—I hate them!" said Phyllis. We softened that darkness. (See page 115.)

Maureen McGovern

Dull eyes and a too strong jaw are transformed with color. (See page 116.)

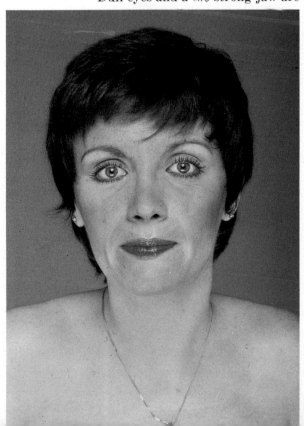
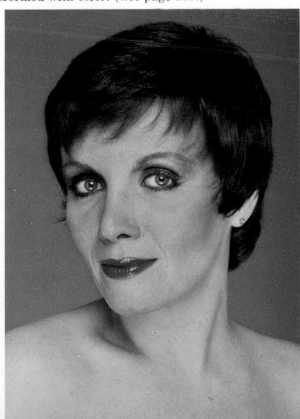

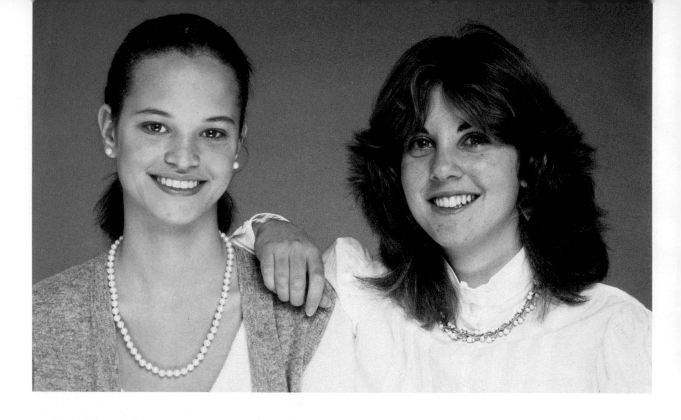

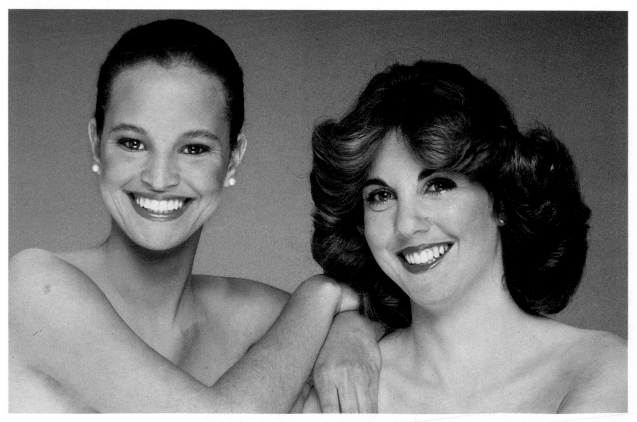

Susan Gross and Nina Pierce

Pallor from late-night studying (and partying) gives way to drama with subtle color added to these college beauties. (See page 115.)

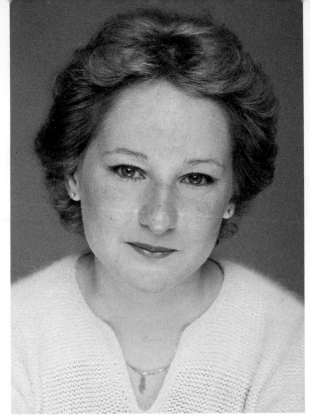
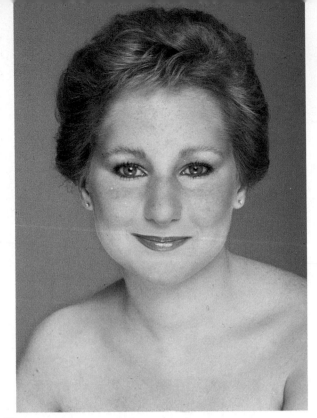

Shelley Bruce

Now, and tomorrow, tomorrow—this star of *Annie* can smile without having her eyes disappear—her pet hate. (See page 117.)

Heather Henderson

Makeup changed the usual adolescent acne and a pleasant face into glowing skin and absolutely knockout beauty. (See page 117.)

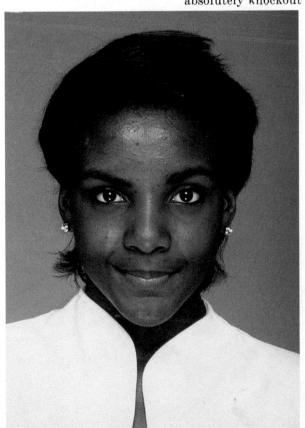
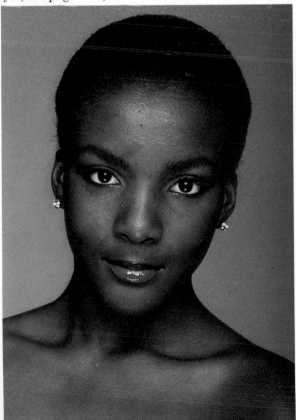

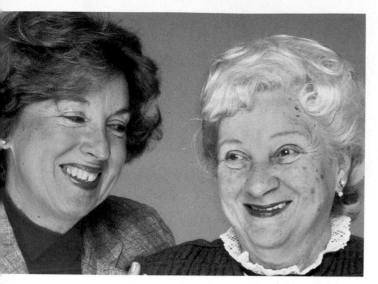
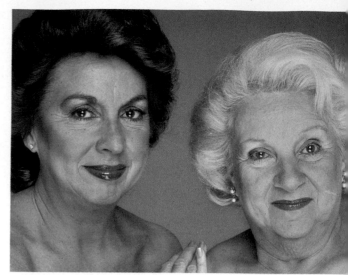

Mildred Hirsch and Lee Bialick

Over-forty doesn't mean under-beautiful. Gorgeous is the word—not old—for my mother and grandmother in makeup. (See page 116.)

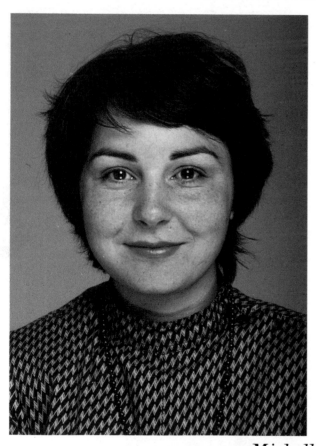
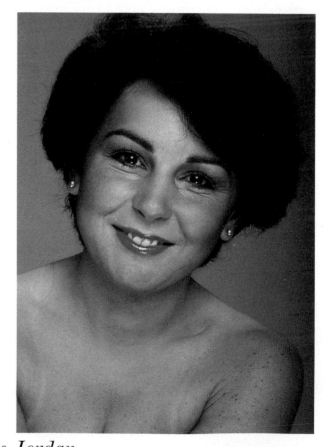

Michelle Jordan

An androgynous face becomes a sexy woman's face with properly applied color. (See page 117.)

IN LIVING COLOR: THE MAKEOVERS EXPLAINED

Ann Reinking	*Problems*	*Solutions*
Star of Broadway's *Dancin'* and of the movie *Annie*.	Too square jawline.	Contour *under* the jawline softened it, and ''parentheses'' contour framing her eyes and cheekbones gave structure to face.
	Low eyebrows.	Brow hairs brushed down, then feathered in on top, to raise brow, after which own brow brushed back up.
	Too little eyeliner on bottom of eye and too little on top.	Eyeliner balanced and concealer under eye highlighted.
	Lips not defined.	Well defined ''bow'' on lips and stronger color.

Elizabeth Hubbard	*Problems*	*Solutions*
Star of the long-running soap opera *The Doctors*.	Thin mouth has tendency to droop and look hard.	Mouth clearly defined and brightly colored, slightly picked up at the corners.
	Pale skin, blond hair makes her ''disappear.''	Beige foundation covers see-through skin. Red rouge color applied in a half-moon line from the end of the nostrils to the hairline and blended.
	Eyes can overpower rest if not strongly balanced in lower face.	Heavy eye makeup in mauve, grey, teal and burgundy widened and accentuated magnificent eyes.
	Nasal lines and blemishes characteristic of fair skin.	Concealer on lines and blemishes, blended and powdered.
	Longish nose.	Contour on sides and tip of nose made it seem shorter.

Carol Lipson	*Problems*	*Solutions*
''Civilian.''	Too harsh ''Cleopatra eyes'' that pointed to every wrinkle.	Softened pencil instead of liquid liner no longer heavily *rings* the eye.
	Too dark makeup base.	Lighter foundation. Muted fuchsia lip color.
	Too red lipstick that clashed with her sky-blue eyes.	

Lizbeth Mackay	*Problems*	*Solutions*
Broadway star of *Crimes of the Heart*.	Endographic skin that shows every blemish.	Meticulous blending of foundation with good coverage conceals blotchiness and redness. Soft sable brush with powder sets foundation.
	A dreary complexion, too pale eyes.	Blue eyes emphasized with shadows in grape, orchid, smoke and denim navy blue.
	Mouth lost in face.	Pure Cupid's bow outlined on Vivien Leigh mouth and lifted a millimeter gave form to nebulous mouth.

Martine Van Hamel	*Problems*	*Solutions*
Prima ballerina of the American Ballet Theatre.	Fleshy, too soft face.	Contour in sideways *V* with point at hairline.
	Eyes seem to get lost.	Khaki eye shadow, fanned out at outer corners, accentuates natural almond shape and conceals hooded lid; heavy mascara and definite eyeliner open up green eyes.
	Wide nose.	Contouring gives aquiline nose (down sides and on tip).
	Blemished skin.	Cream foundation provides greater coverage.

Dominique Singer	*Problems*	*Solutions*
"Civilian."	Sallow, dull complexion.	Olive-based foundation to zip up the color. Contour shading would have been overkill on her already prominent bone structure, so red-red rouge and lipstick were enough to give her face new color vitality.
	Tired-looking eyes.	Heavy eye makeup in the brown and russet family sparked exoticism in her eyes, and concealer erased the heavy, dark under-eye circles.

Phyllis Newman	*Problems*	*Solutions*
Actress, writer, conversationalist, and giggler extraordinaire.	Dark circles under the eyes.	Two layers of concealer on under-eye circles.
	Sallow, washed-out skin.	Foundation evens out color and blusher enlivens it.
	Lines and wrinkles in the outer eye corners.	Concealer on lines.
	Dark lidded eyes give tired look.	Instead of fighting dark lids, go with a deep purple shadow: the brown shadow she'd been wearing matched her eyes and caused them to retract. Thin lash-line instead of thick lets lashes stand out against lid.

Susan Gross and Nina Pierce	*Problems*	*Solutions*
Brown University roommates.	SUE has fragile, transparent skin of natural blond.	Good makeup base, to even out skin tone and conceal visible blemishes.
	Pallor and puffiness from late night study.	Concealer to mute puffs (applied only on line of demarcation and not directly *on* puff).
	Soft eyes are not accentuated enough.	Wonderful eyes made more wonderful with subtle peach, grape and smoke shadows and an aqua eyeliner to emphasize green-grey eyes. Color is minimally applied on young face but color is definitely needed.
	NINA has too prominent forehead.	A mixed heritage has endowed Nina with the bones and facial structure of a high fashion model: forehead shaded with contour to soften it.
	Eyes that droop very slightly.	Almond-shaped eyes tipped with smoky shading slightly up instead of down. Dark crayon inside eyeledge gave mysterious profundity.
	Sallow skin tone.	Light base gave life to skin. What a face!

Maureen McGovern	*Problems*	*Solutions*
Singer, actress.	Too strong jaw.	A semi-triangle of contour was brushed on with the point resting at center of hairline and triangle arms moving on a slant to temples. From the temple points, contour powder was brushed in another slant under the cheekbones, which gave more width to the jaw and muted the chin point.
	"Washed out" eyes.	Maureen's magnificent eyes were accentuated by heavy application of charcoal under lower lid and marine blue inside lower lid.
	Undefined mouth.	Clear lip liner application (drawn, then blended) gives definite and dramatic mouth. Rosy lip color and gloss, added together, finish the newly sensual mouth.

Mildred Hirsch and Lee Bialick	*Problems*	*Solutions*
They're my mother and grandmother, both gorgeous and with many of the same problems.	Dry skin and liver spots.	Cream foundation to equalize dry skin pigment. An extra foundation base on my grandmother to mute liver spots.
	Neck jowls.	Contour applied in horizontal rather than diagonal line to "cut" faces in half and bring attention up to eyes. Contour paints out sag under neck and jowls.
	Grandmother's "pink" eye look.	Teal crayon on wet ledge of grandmother's lower lash-line takes away pinkness.
	Wrinkles.	Eye interest detracts from face wrinkles. Note how "dropping" the inner corner with teal and "lifting" the outer corner with pewter gave my grandmother a more interesting, almond-shaped eye. Eye shadows: Pewter, orchid and teal on grandmother. Smoke, rose, khaki and marine green crayon on wet ledge for mother.

Shelley Bruce
Star of *Annie*.

Problems
Deep-set eyelids give an eye-overhang that makes Shelley's eyes "disappear" when she smiles.

Solutions
Light tan shadow on the lids made them more dramatic (darkness hides, lightness brings out).

under-eye concealer applied, not for circles or blemishes but to make the frontal bone more prominent.

Brushing brows up gave more room for space and color.

Shadows: 1) Gold frost, 2) Rose frost, 3) Light brown, 4) Lime sorbet.

Lashes curled to further "open" eyes.

Problems
Round face, pointed chin.

Solutions
Contour applied to sculpt bones.

Problems
Colorless skin.

Solutions
Cream rouge on forehead and chin when blended gives rosy blush to skin.

Heather Henderson
Student.

Problems
Adolescent acne.

Solutions
Sandstone-color base covers pimples. Slightly lighter base used instead of concealer because concealer too light for Heather's dark skin. Base is also lighter in texture— better for adolescent skin.

Problems
Acid in lips which causes lip color to turn darker.

Solutions
Base applied over lips before adding color.

Problems
Masque of lightness around eyes.

Solutions
Base used as concealer again (in a lighter shade).

Problems
Dull eyes.

Solutions
Gold frost under brow, deep purple on lid, deep smoke in outer corner, khaki in inner corner, marine blue inside lower lid and charcoal under lid brought these magnificent sloe-eyes to life.

Michelle Jordan
Advertising executive.

Problems
Rounded face makes Michelle look like a cute kid.

Solutions
Heavy contour under cheekbones to carve out facial interest.

Problems
Almond-shaped eyes lost in too round face.

Solutions
Heavy mascara, mauve frost under brow, pewter on lid, grape in outer corner, burgundy towards nose wake up eyes.

Problems
Sallow skin.

Solutions
Cinnamon-colored base and pink blusher patted in "parentheses" around eyes and up onto forehead make skin luscious.

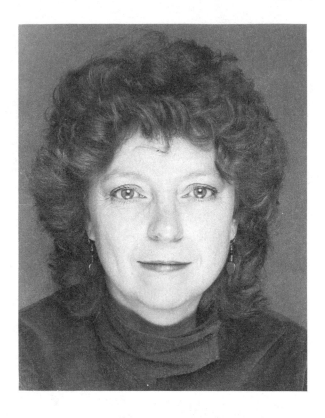

SKIN

Often it's the light, translucent skin that gives the most problems. Every vein and blemish peers out of this sheer canvas and the face takes on a flaky, pasty look. As these women age, lines seem like crevices, and blotchiness and whiteness can make someone almost disappear.

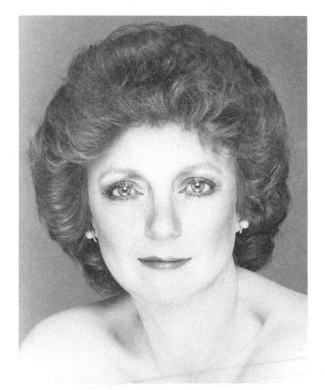

Jan Goodwin

She's the executive editor of *The Ladies' Home Journal,* and being very English, it's no surprise that she has the traditional peaches-and-cream English skin. Her fabulous red hair tends to make this fair skin look somewhat blotchy in contrast. It looked wonderful with a porcelain cream-base which evened out the many tones. An earth shade of golden apricot blusher and a berry rouge gave interest and shading to the sheer skin, and concealer both under and over the base toned down a nose which had a tendency toward pinkness. Earth tones on her eyes, gold smoke on the lid, pewter in the corner, yellow crayon under the brow and brown velvet on the outer lid were wonderful stages for her ''bedroom'' eyes of forest green. A full peaked mouth in a bright melon gave additional contrast and interest to her skin.

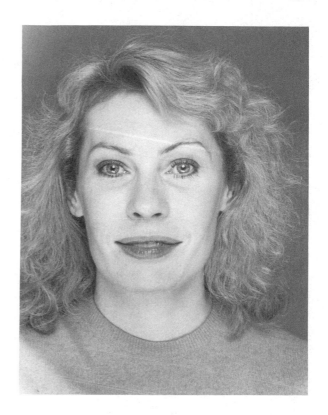

Hope Stansbury

A stunning blond who looks like she walked out of an F. Scott Fitzgerald novel, she has translucent skin that makes her almost an invisible woman. Lines and under-eye puffs, common with this kind of skin, make her tired looking. Concealer under the eyes and carried out to the temples over a smooth foundation provided a skin without a break between the eyes and the rest of the face. Light powdering disguised hollows under the eyes. Strong color accentuated a wonderfully aquiline face and a perfect mouth, and great bones suddenly emerged with contour color. Heavy, heavy mascara brought attention to bland eyes, and Hope, a vision in muted mauves, grapes, purples and sherry satin, was transformed from dishwatery to dynamic.

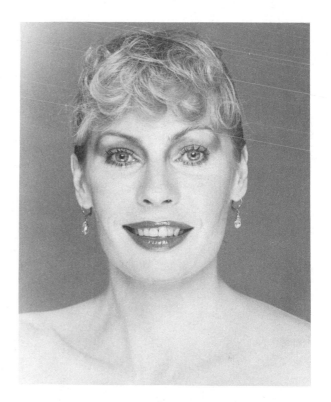

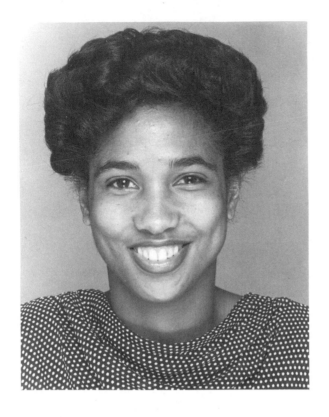

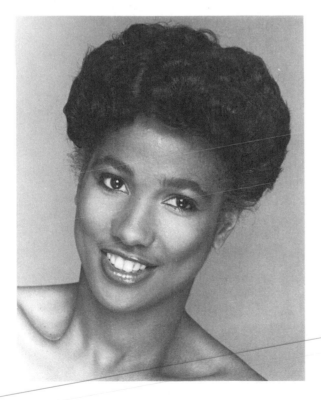

Lorna Dawkins

Aspiring model, receptionist at a major New York publishing house, Lorna has the multi-pigmented skin of so many black women. Because a lighter foundation (which I generally advocate) did not seem to work for her skin, I tried a slightly darker-than-her-natural-skin-tone color and it was perfect! Every rule has an exception. Some dark shading over her lip was another skin color problem—solved by drawing a *very* definite mouth line with lip liner, the line blended and then luscious color applied. Under-eye circles on the skin were erased by using a lighter foundation shade in place of concealer.

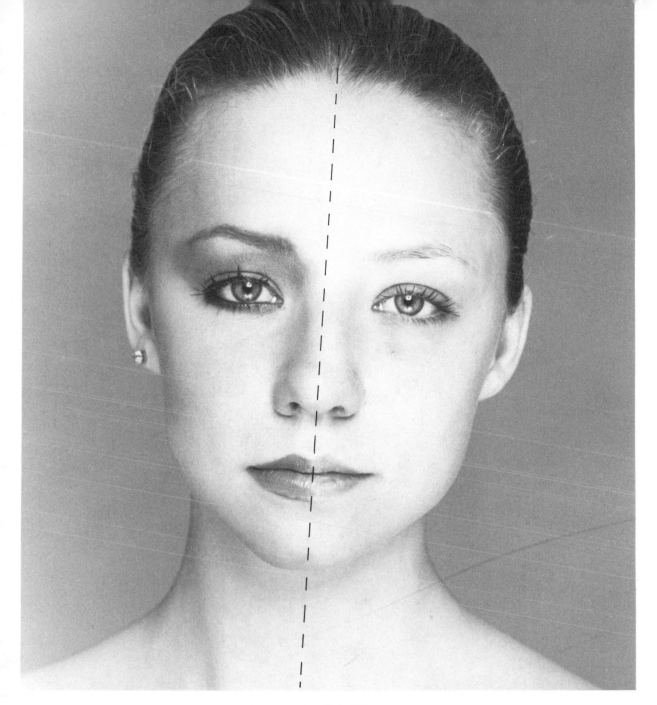

Amanda McKerrow

HALF FACES

It's easy to see the wonder of makeup when you can check out a *before* and an *after* on the same face. AMANDA McKERROW and LISA deRIBERE are two ballet dancers with the American Ballet Theatre.

*

Notice the *before* part of Amanda's face. It's pale, there are puffs and circles under the eyes, she looks tired and jowly. Now consider the *after* half of the face. What has emerged with makeup is a striking blond, more alive, more beautiful, more ready to play the part of a romantic heroine.

*

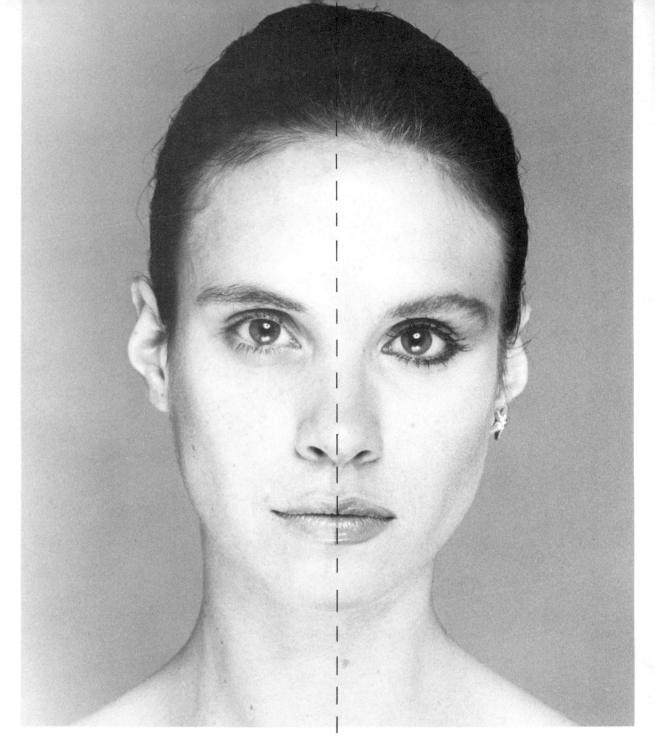

Lisa deRibere

Ignore the made-up portion of Lisa's face. Her eyes don't shine, her mouth disappears, her face looks gaunt not exotic. Now look at the *after* side: A stunner appears with limpid eyes, sculptured contours, *Swan Lake* elegance.

*

Don't tell me that makeup doesn't perform wonders.

5*

Special People, Special Places

AN UNDER-EIGHTEEN SKIN CARE AND MAKEUP GUIDE

Little girl makeup kits sold better than Atari television games last Christmas. The inescapable truth is that, along with their mothers and grandmas, most females from a very young age care about how they appear to others. *Want* to look pretty. *Want* to feel glamorous. And glamour has everything to do with careful makeup and skin care. It's a fact of life. If it's true that in America we tend to go somewhat overboard on the notion that beauty comes out of bottles, still we have learned the best ways to present that beauty and to preserve it for the longest years.

The key is to start young. It really is. The beauty rituals you adapt at sixteen are for your whole life. The skin care regimens you learn at thirteen will stand you in good stead when you're sixty. The way you look before you're twenty often presages the face you'll show to the world all your life. Why not start out right? I'm not suggesting that you in-

struct your eleven-year-old on the nuances of contouring; I only say that if you teach your eleven-year-old how to give herself a facial (the art of cleanliness is ageless and timeless), then when it comes time for the contouring, she'll do it expertly and finely and easily because she won't have to fight the pimples to find the cheekbones.

FIRST COMES HEALTHY SKIN!

Start at the beginning. And I really mean At The Beginning. When a young mother bundles up her toddler for the fresh-air walk on the coldest winter day, the baby is often snowsuited so heavily, her little arms stick out at right angles. She's toasty warm, that baby—everywhere but on her face. And, oh, that little face. Made ruddy and healthy looking by the cold, it is often only a victim of wind- or sunburn. The rosy cheeks her mother admires set the stage for weakened capillary structure, and when she's twenty she'll wonder why she has all those spidery little veins bursting so easily in her face. A light layer of cream or Vaseline would provide an easy protective armor against hot sun or cold wind, but in our society no one thinks about skin care for three-year-olds. They should.

Before you know it, she's eight. And ripe for imitating of mommy. Make a game of daily face cleansing. It's a time for sharing and learning and starting habits that will give her the finest skin in town when she's twenty. The whole thing starts with face washing—yours and hers. While you use a cleanser, this is the only time in her life when she can gleefully lather up with soap—a mild, transparent glycerine soap (Original Formula Neutrogena is a good bet). You both lather up, you don't yell when she splashes water on the floor and you both revel in a clean face.

Two rules for the very young soap-users:

* Your daughter must learn to rinse off all traces of the soap. Even if this involves a whole lot of water-logged towels, it's important.
* The soap is to be gently lathered on—not massaged into the skin with the fingers or any device.

A note about bubble baths, as long as we're talking soap: I strongly advise against them. They're fun but dangerous. Bubble bath is not made from true soap but from synethetic detergents—the kind of stuff that shampoo and laundry soap are made from. Pediatricians report too many cases of skin irritation and urinary tract infections which are directly traceable to bubble baths.

After the cleaning comes the creaming. There's nothing more fun for an eight-year-old than sharing a bit of her mother's soothing creams. Her own skin can be surprisingly dry. In fact, getting her her very own moisturizing creams in her own jars, to be kept in her own beauty corner, is a really loving thing to do. Putting a thin layer of cream on the face is more than a beauty lesson: It's a lesson in environmental protection. Lubriderm, which can be purchased in any drugstore, is just fine for your little girl and it's even finer if you put it into one of your own, fancier cream jars before you give it to her.

A little cream protection from the elements, cold or sun, goes a very long way. You might also, at this age, begin teaching your young daughter about taking the sun in small doses: To overindulge in the sun's ultraviolet rays has a cumulative effect and current research has it that skin cancer and wrinkling can actually have their roots in the too-much, too-soon exposure of the eight- or nine-year-old child.

Setting aside time each day for skin care starts a habit that's hard to break. As soon as a kid can copy, she can begin.

Now, we get down to business. Setting the stage is one thing. It's mashed potatoes compared to what has to come next, which is *serious* skin care. I don't want to imply that serious means hard or unpleasant; on the contrary, it can be enormously enjoyable. The adolescent and often the preadolescent —ten-, eleven- or twelve-year-olds—has no-kidding-around skin problems to deal with now. This is *sturm und drang* time. On the one hand, adolescent skin can be at its very zenith. No sags, bags, wrinkles, broken capillaries have yet made an appearance; its texture is soft, its color is delightful. On the other hand, becoming a sexual person has its down side, because with the onset of puberty the hormones go full steam ahead. Oil glands go berserk, grow monstrously and begin to

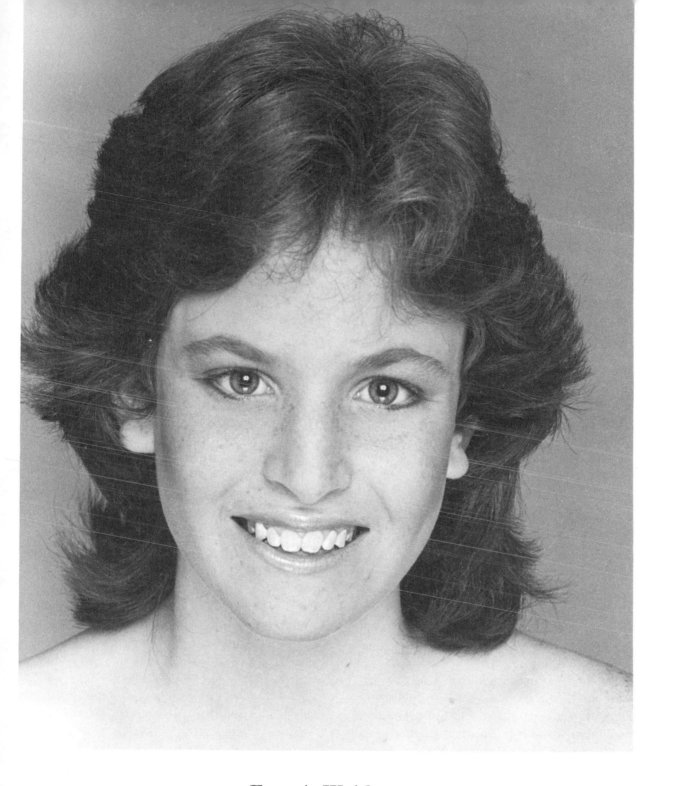

Francie Weisler:

Sweet Sixteen and Beautiful!

pour out junk, which in turn clogs newly thickened pores. Result: zitsville. It's very depressing to have a pus-pimple on the tip of your nose before the prom. It could make a person very cranky. Your teenager is beginning to be aware that her menstrual cycle sometimes acts as announcement of a skin breakout. She's seeing a *preventable* pattern: if she takes extra cleansing care the week *before* her period, she can often break the cycle of period-pimples. Her skin care is not copy-cat stuff any more; she's a woman in her own right and if she's to avoid the pock-marks and lifetime scarring that comes from adolescent breakouts, she has to give skin care a big part in her life. These directions, therefore, are for her.

A DAILY CLEANSING SCHEDULE FOR THE TEENAGER

CLEANSING At least twice daily and three times is even better! This should be done *not* with medicated cleansers which are worse than worthless because they are (1) irritating (they're often detergent-based) and (2) frauds (the medication doesn't stay on the face long enough to do any good). And *not* with soap: throw out the little girl soap; you're a big girl now and should never let it touch your big girl skin again.

It should be done with a gentle and thorough cleansing cream or lotion (they're the same except creams are solid and lotions are liquid). I particularly recommend a water-soluble product for adolescent skin because it rinses off with water and doesn't leave a film residue—a big plus for skins that are plagued with an outpouring of oil. A gentle cleanser that many of my young clients recommend is Winthrop Laboratories' pHisoderm which lathers well, is good for most skin types and rinses off in hard or soft water.

FRESHENER Use two or three times daily. The oily adolescent skin is the only skin that can really benefit from an *alcohol*-based freshener, which should never be used after, say, age eighteen. The alcohol can be very drying to older skins, but adolescents benefit wonderfully from the alcohol's ability to remove oil, dirt and sebum deposits—as well as any traces of cleanser that may be left from a non-water-soluble cleanser. One good alcohol-based freshener is Clinique's Clarifying Lotion 2. If you don't mind the rather strong odor, plain witch hazel (Dickinson's is one reputable brand) cleans very well and is quite inexpensive. If you have very dry skin (a rarity for teenagers), don't use an alcohol-based freshener. If you have the usual adolescent oiliness, *wipe* the alcohol freshener on with a saturated pad—don't just pat it on, which removes nothing. This freshener should also tighten your pores, provide a cooling, soothing sensation and make you look glowing!

After using freshener, I always advise my clients to follow with a *cold* water rinse which removes much of the alcohol from the skin. Of course, if you use a freshener without any alcohol (like my own brand), the rinse is unnecessary.

MOISTURIZER In the morning, before applying makeup, and in the evening, before bed. Next to cleansing, the adolescent skin needs moisture most. Because a moisturizer should be made up predominantly of water and not oil, it will not make your skin more oily, despite what you've heard. Just use your common sense: I've heard colleagues advise teenagers to spread a thin film of mineral or baby oil over their skin. That's terrible! It's like bringing coals to Newcastle—adding oil to an already oil-burdened skin. But moisturizer is very different. It's a protective barrier between you and the makeup and between you and the environment which includes smoke, soot, wind, sun. Apply it on a *damp* skin (Evian mineral water in a spray bottle is nice to dampen skin). Suggestions? Shiseido puts a good moisturizer out for very oily skin and Elizabeth Arden's Active Day Protecting Moisture-Cream is popular with young people with dryer skins. Despite the advertising geared to the young market, many of my clients have been dissatisfied with Bonne Bell moisturizers which they say feel very greasy.

EYE CREAMS   If anyone wants to sell you, a teenager, an eye cream, tell them thanks but no thanks: Teenagers don't need eye cream.

A WEEKLY MAINTENANCE SCHEDULE FOR THE TEENAGER

EXFOLIATION   Once or twice weekly. The nails, an extension of skin, have to be trimmed regularly, and so does the skin. Removing the dead skin cells that build up drastically reduces the number of blackheads and whiteheads and other Uglies that are prevalent on adolescent skin. I recommend a skin-peeling cream because cream is mild and does the job wonderfully, but for this exfoliating process many teenagers prefer the scrub-type cleansers like Dorothy Gray's Cleansing Grains or Stiefel Laboratories' Brasivol Lathering Scrub Cleanser for Acne. I suppose you can get away with using them without doing too much damage if you just gently massage them into the skin for no more than fifteen seconds at a time (never scrub, no matter what the directions say), and wipe off with a warm cloth. Scrub-cleansers should never be used after you're twenty: They tend to break capillar-

ies and damage skin. But, whatever you use, as a teenager, you must exfoliate regularly—that is, remove the scales and flakes that are invisibly gathering on the surface layer of the skin.

EJECTION   Once or twice weekly; three times if your skin is really bad. Even though it may be hard to sit still without talking for ten minutes or so, you should follow the exfoliation process with a facial masque. It's probably even more important for you than for your mother. It's *you* who needs the tightening action of that masque because instead of applying dermatologist-prescribed medicines on your face to get rid of impurities, the simple constriction pushes impurities to the surface—often all that's needed. If you absolutely hate the feeling of the full masque, you can masque-up on problem areas. Say only your forehead is prone to terrible pimples: Only apply the masque there. After ten minutes, wipe off with a warm washcloth. A good product to try is Orlane's Ligne Active Masque Bleu, which is particularly nice for oily skin.

And remember: Your skin must get worse before it gets better. When you first begin exfoliating and ejection, your skin will break out the next day. It has to. The bad stuff is coming out and you're setting the stage for maintenance. After that first breakout episode, except for rare occasions when there's a lot of oily buildup, your skin will not respond so dramatically to the weekly schedule. Try to do it the day before you have nothing to do, for safety's sake.

THE LAST WORD—NO-NO'S

∗ Avoid fooling with your face—touching the face to feel for pimples, squeezing blackheads, sitting with the face in the hand. It *all* promotes dirt on the face and more trouble.

* Avoid high alcohol-based fresheners, high oil-based products.

* Avoid sharing makeup with your best friend, especially eye makeup: It's a wonderful way to spread infection.

Makeup for Minors: Ten Steps to Dynamite!

If you are old enough to wear makeup, you're old enough to do it right. Only you can decide what look you want and at what age to start creating it with color, but one thing's for sure: applying makeup is a *learned* skill which improves with practice. The art of makeup for the very young depends on having a *light* touch. Colors from a box and a jar can make you look more lovely—and they can also, when used with overkill, make you look like a toddler who fell into her mother's makeup drawer. Too much of a good thing can give a heavy-handed, harsh and cheap look. Here's a step-by-step guide for the teenager who wants to perfect her makeup techniques. Natural beauty requires work!

First, set the stage for practice: Have a soda ready for the times when your hand slips and your eyeliner ends up on your nose. Have your materials all set out in front of you, as an artist does with her paints. Have plenty of cotton pads and cleanser ready for mistakes.

Now, go! (Naturally, your face is *Absolutely clean* . . . right?)

1. Start with a clean face: use a lemon or regular cleanser. With a clean cotton pad, apply a freshener, particularly around the nose to discourage the oilies.

2. Apply a thin layer of moisturizer if you plan to wear any makeup at all on your face. It acts as a barrier between your pores and the foundation or blusher.

3. Spot the lightest of bases on your cheekbones, nose and forehead in "measles" dots. A see-through glaze is quite nice for young skin. Blend very well and never pile on the foundation in the hope it will hide your blemishes. It won't.

4. Lightly apply blusher to the apples of your cheeks and carry it through to the hairline.

5. Brush up brows with a toothbrush that has been lightly sprayed with hair spray, for a "feathery" wide open look.

6. Curl your lashes—be careful to open the curler before you remove it. Apply the first eye shadow under the brow (a pearlized pink or a mauve is a nice choice). This will open up your eye. Apply the second shadow on your lid; don't try to match your eyes but pick up a glint in your skin tone or clothing (try peach, light grey, toast). Shadows are always in powder, applied with a brush and blended well.

7. A brown or grey crayon under the lower lashes, smudged softly and only applied halfway across, will enlarge eyes. For really special evenings, you might try a light green or blue crayon *in* the lower wet ledge of the eye to make the whites of your eyes look whiter. Be careful you don't poke the crayon in your eye!

8. Mascara time! Go wild with black no matter what color your lashes are: Hold the mascara wand vertically and apply the color from the inner corner to the outer corner in a horizontal sweep on upper and lower lashes.

9. A colored gloss for your lips can be applied with a brush or your little finger.

10. Finish off with a light dusting of translucent powder.

BEST FACE FORWARD: OVER FORTY

They've written you off haven't they, and it's damned annoying. Wear less makeup after forty, they tell you, or else you'll look hard and even older. Pay more attention to spiritual values, perhaps, is the unwritten message, and forget about the way you look when the wrinkles come, because you can never compete with the starlets.

Garbage. There is nothing more gorgeous, more appealing, than a ripened woman who has grown accustomed to her face. She isn't trying to compete with starlets when she skillfully brings out the seasoned sensuality she's earned. And the way she does that is with more, not less, makeup—more artfully applied. Because she's fighting gravity and loss of moisture, she has to compensate with better products—and she can't skimp on coverage. You know, it takes very little makeup to look like a streetwalker and a great deal of makeup to look natural. It does take time, though, and some expense. You simply cannot get away with a dab of blusher anymore. Your carefully acquired-through-the-years sense of style and beauty can't stop at the neck. I know too many women who spend a fortune on a new pair of boots or a great coat and then walk around with the same, tired face, because they've been brainwashed to believe that makeup should be drastically reduced after forty. Listen—I've seen Sophia Loren without her makeup and believe me, she doesn't look so hot.

Beauty does *not* belong to the young. Pretty paint and wise skin care can transform dull maturity into *great* sophistication. If you're over forty, and your unimaginative cousin tries to shame you into an Early Rocking Chair style, say something shocking to her and put on a little more shading! It'll do

wonders for your personal image, not to mention your sexuality. Despite what the "purist" life-destroyers say, your theme song should not be resignation, but something like, "If They Could See Me Now . . ."

First of all, some general advice. Stay away from the old lady colors of mauve and black: They do nothing to wake up your face and they tend to dampen your personality also. And go over your habits which are hard to kill: the one of matching everything, for instance. That's aging, and when your nails, bag and shoes match your eye shadow everyone knows you came of age forty years ago when matching was the vogue. Throw out the thick pan-sticks and the no-glide lipsticks that have been cluttering your medicine cabinet for twelve years. That's all right, go ahead and *waste* them even if they look perfectly new!!! Vow to start this week of your life with a fresh new set of makeup. Vow to experiment with your face and try at least one new look this week. Go ahead—add another shadow on those lids—it'll do wonders for you if you remember to blend it with the other three. It's never too late to coax any age skin into stunning beauty.

Clean Up Your Act!

There's no question that improper cleansing techniques can aggravate the skin's sensitivity, and granular cleansers, irritating soaps and harsh sponges can make your over-forty skin a mess. You need to use the most gentle makeup remover you can find, which you will tissue off, along with the dirt and makeup, every night. Soap products almost inevitably leave a filmy residue on the skin, no matter how much you rinse, and that *dries* —something you never need, particularly in middle age. You're experiencing a real decline in oil production and your face looks it (the skin is tougher and the pores seem larger), and it feels it (it's very vulnerable to irritation). For the latter reason, heat applied through facial sauna, very hot water or hot towels is to be avoided like the plague.

Consider the water you use: if it's very hard or if it has a high mineral content it will not rinse and cleanse well. Bottled, distilled water was practically invented for you to rinse with as well as to drink!

If you've never exfoliated before (shame!), now you really have no choice. Age brings an accumulation of dead skin-cells which, left to their own devices, give a coarse, thick appearance. The dead surface skin *must* be removed if you're not to look like the alligator lady at the circus. Loofah sponges and Buf-Puf products are too rough and may cause great irritation to your newly sensitive skin, so be sure to follow the directions given in the Skin-Care Two-Step (see Chapter 2). The only places where you can use a pumice stone or loofah sponge safely are on the heels and elbows, where cellular buildup comes on very strong. (If you have a particular problem with cracked elbows and heels, wrap them in Saran Wrap overnight! I'm not kidding: Exfoliating heels and elbows by putting a layer of Vaseline on the area and gift-wrapping the whole business by taping closed the edges makes for the softest, moistest heels and elbows in the morning. Plastic bags on the feet work as well as Saran Wrap.) Whatever you do to your elbows and heels, you should be meticulous in exfoliating your face about three times weekly after forty years of age.

Moisturizing is the name of the game now, even if you've never paid much attention to it before. Water it from the outside with non-

oil-based moisturizers and—I know I'm courting controversy here—oil it from the inside. Despite what you've heard and read, it's madness to eliminate all oils and fats from the diet. The latest medical thinking has it that eating cholesterol-based products hardly counts at all after fifty, and much medical evidence is pointing to the fact that what you eat doesn't contribute in an important way to cholesterol buildup, anyway. You can even avoid the whole controversy by sticking to polyunsaturated products like safflower oil in your cooking and even as a diet supplement in the form of about a tablespoon of oil a day—cold turkey. Why? Because it helps your skin to better utilize protein and replenishes lost oils in the aging body. Ask any veterinarian what is prescribed for a dog whose skin is dry and flaking: a tablespoon of oil in its Alpo! The Airedale's skin and hair take on an amazing gloss and vitality. If it's good for your dog, why stint on yourself? Check with your doctor if you don't believe me . . . but *do* check! Speaking of oil, the over fifty-year-old model Carmen puts the oil from a vitamin E capsule in her bath at night and often smooths the liquid right on her face. Another moisturizer she likes is an application of half milk, half water under her makeup.

Lack of sleep; heavy alcohol, drug or tobacco use and air pollution can be murder on older skin. I'm not telling you to move if you live in Cleveland, but don't step out of your door without a protective agent on your face.

SHED LIGHT ON THE MATTER

Look, no one should make up in the closet, but it's even more important for you to make up in the light in which you'll be seen than for anyone else. What's important is to see what everyone else will be seeing—even if

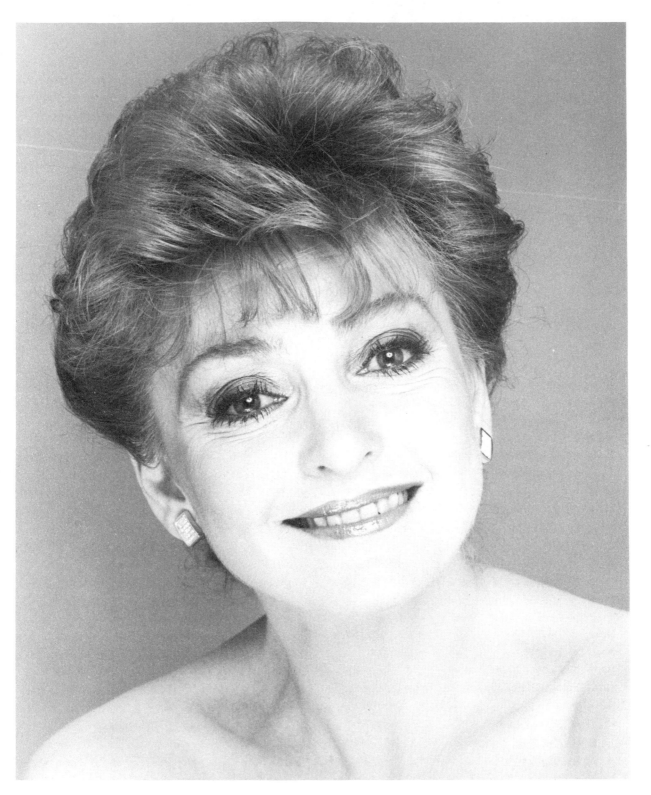

Lee Ducat

Founder of the Juvenile Diabetes Foundation, over 40 and fantastic.

those wrinkles are tough to face. Outside, you'll need a lightweight cream for the coverage. Inside, perhaps you can get away with a lighter liquid. Fluorescent lighting can age faces so check yourself out in a fluorescent light to compensate in the makeup colors. And although I believe that older women must wear more not less makeup, the one exception is if you plan to be in the bright sunlight all day: Unless you're really expert at applying colors, a lot of makeup looks garish in sunlight—even if it's well blended.

Grown-Up Beauty

THE FOUNT OF GROWN-UP BEAUTY It's the foundation, and it's probably the single most important aspect of the over-forty makeup. It's terrific, in many ways, to be mature and seasoned, but one of the not-so-terrific aspects to seasoning are the infinite colors of the facial spices. Small brownish speckling, uneven skin tone, broken capillaries and liver spots can wreck the most careful makeup application.

Liver spots have nothing to do with the liver and everything to do with the way they *resemble* liver. Flat, brown marks, they appear on people over fifty and are aggravated by sun exposure. Bleaching has negligible results, cryosurgery (freezing with liquid nitrogen or carbon dioxide) causes them to lighten, but this should only be done by a qualified medical doctor. I suggest foundation which, artfully applied, minimizes them. While foundation cannot cover completely, it can surely blend and tone down most all skin irregularities. Avoid thick, heavy bases and powder with color. They tend to accent wrinkles, leaving residues in them that make a fine line look like the San Andreas Fault. Lighter-color bases tend to wash out those lines better than deeper-color bases.

Cream is preferable to liquid for the over-forty makeup because of its greater coverage, and the color should be a shade *lighter* than your own skin because dark will only stain and emphasize the liver spots. Dot on with a Q-Tip and blend with your fingers: A sponge only eats up your foundation and is very unclean; besides—who is *that* meticulous about rinsing it out? Blend very well into the neck, under the chin, around and behind ears and don't forget the earlobes. *Avoid* cake makeup: It always looks mask-like. Now, don't judge your face by your foundation: If it looks a little chalky, wait till you add the contour and the blusher and the rouge before you race for a darker color.

CONCEALER God gave you crow's-feet and eye bags, but he was also merciful enough to provide concealer. It's your best friend. Use it. On liver spots, burst capillaries, shadows around the mouth—in fact, on every blemish that the woman over forty hates, concealer conceals, minimizes, even reshapes. Don't rub it in—you'll lose the concealing effect if you do. If, after softly blending in the area, you still note a lighter area that stands out too much, don't get hysterical. By the time you finish applying your contour, rouge, blusher and translucent powder, it shouldn't show up.

EYE MAKEUP First of all, the trick is to try to prevent more crow's-feet and under-eye lines from appearing, and the best way to do that is to use an *eye cream* every night. I have heard some colleagues recommend a lightweight eye oil to be applied over makeup several times a day in an effort to keep these areas constantly moist, but I really think that's overkill. What's more, it will make you the greasiest looking over-forty in town. There are some line-softening sticks containing lanolin or castor oil that come in a lipstick-like container and that are created to be used over makeup, but unless you have a serious dryness problem, I'd stick with the night cream.

Now, for the makeup. *Concentrate* on great eyes: They draw attention away from the rest of the face and eyes never age.

The first rule of thumb is *more, more mascara*. You can't wear too much and it should always be black. Today's mascara wands are almost guaranteed to give a perfect application, and mascara should always be applied holding the wand vertically and then brushing it against the eyelashes in a horizontal sweep from eye corner to outer lash: This is the best way to thicken and darken without clumping.

Wispy eyebrows are devastatingly aging. Sticking to the natural brow-line, feather in your brows with a brush-on brow powder and a sharp brush.

Eye pencils are a must for the woman over forty: They should be soft and almost creamy so the color slides on easily, and the eyeliner should line the lashes not quite a quarter of an inch below. Always softly smudge the liner (dark greys and blues look fine) above and below the lash-line to make the eye seem clear and limpid as a mountain stream. A dark pencil *inside* the upper and lower rim also lends clarity and focus.

Experiment with eye shadows, but never use frosted colors which only highlight lines and wrinkles. Liquid creams are only for the very young of face (not heart, necessarily), because they tend to coagulate, get oily and generally draw attention to imperfections. Your (and everybody's) best bet is the versatile powders. Soft, dusky shades over the eyelids with deeper violets and greys at the outer corners and lighter colors blended up to the brow are effective for "opening" the eye.

An absolute must for the mature woman is her eyelash curler. It brings the lashes up and over the puffier eyelids, practically can-

celing them out. Be sure you use the curler *before* you put on mascara to avoid taking out half the lashes.

NECKLINES Sagging or loose necks and multiple chins present a common makeup problem for the over-forty woman. Try using a slightly darker foundation on this kind of neck, making sure you blend well into your facial foundation. Brush on contour under the chin, over the whole neck area, to effectively "erase" the problem area.

LIPSTICKS AND LINERS Lip liner is essential in the over-forty makeup. It gives a definite shape to a droopy mouth and it prevents the lipstick from bleeding into the fine lines that are developing around your mouth. Use a burgundy shade which most closely approximates your natural lip color and blend the liner in softly so you don't have an obvious line around your mouth. Lip color should be brighter, more intense. A muddy brown lipstick is aging and unattractive. Gloss can be applied by brush *with* the lip color for a translucent look, or gently applied to the bottom lip with a fingertip.

THE PARENTHESIS BLUSH Soft puffs of powder blusher in a rosy or amber tone, swept from the outer center of the cheekbone, up and around the temples and over the brow, look terrific on older women. The soft touch of gentle color does sparkly and radiant things to the eyes and upper face. Blusher in a parenthesis shape actually frames the eyes and draws attention away from the lower part of the face.

COLOR We're talking about contour, blusher, cream rouge and eye shadows.

Contour: always, always in a brick-y, earthy shade. Nothing else.
Cream Rouge: avoid orange like crazy. As you age, your teeth tend to lose some of their pristine whiteness and orange on your face makes them look yellow. Also avoid school-

girl pink—it's plain silly on you. Deep corals, deep pinks, deep reds are nicest. Your blusher and rouge should pick up the tones of your lip color. And remember to dab a bit of color on the face wherever there's natural color, like the forehead, earlobes, chin and nose tip.

Blusher: soft burgundies, rusts, corals to carry out the tones of the rouge you choose. Blusher must be gently powdered over rouge if rouge is to last more than ten minutes, and cheek color is *vital* in the forty-plus makeup.

Lipstick: dark browns or maroons are awful and aging. Bright reds, *strong* colors are most effective on older women. As the skin ages, it loses some of its tone, life and, sometimes, color. Brightness on the mouth wakes it up. Think rich, *opulent* colors; eschew wishy-washy.

Eye Colors: anything garish is harsh. Your eye colors should be soft blues, murky greys, chinchilla browns (lighter than earth brown), deep sea-greens. Aqua, golds, sky blue, pinks are for the under-twenty crowd. Brunettes look fine with dark plums and smoky grey shadows; fairer skins with auburns.

Foundations: avoid anything with a yellowish cast because that will make you look sallow. Soft peach or pink undertones in foundation tend to warm up your face with a healthy glow.

Crucial tip about frosteds: Frosted anything yells for attention. Don't put frosted products on crow's-feet, tiny wrinkles, crepey eyelids, unless you love them and want to show them off.

What's a color wash? Something nice. They're nonoily liquids and gels, and they give a delicate, transparent tint of color. Over a tan, they're dynamite!

What's the most important thing? It's blending. You need more, not less makeup as you age, but you also need to blend, blend, blend with a fat brush and translucent powder.

Finally, your age gives you license to be creative. I'm not talking about Early Halloween effects, but a woman who is unique and creative in other respects can have fun with makeup also! I love to see an older woman with wonderful skin paint her lips deeply, passionately red and leave her skin pale. Or a woman with extraordinary eyes doing a garden of greens in mint, olive and emerald, well blended. You have to have courage and the personality to go with it, but creating *effects* that are dramatic has nothing to do with age. Good taste and high style are timeless.

SKIN CARE AND MAKEUP FOR THE BIG WOMAN

There's a part of the population which has always been studiously ignored in beauty and skin care books and that's because, up to now, the myth had it that heavy women (1) didn't spend much time or money on beauty and (2) even if they did, it wouldn't help. Now along with women's and black liberation another segment of the national population is asking for equality, and that is the thirty million American women who are size sixteen and over. Do you know that over 30 percent of the adult female population of America is overweight?

The heavy woman cares about looking terrific, and what's more, she can look sensual, trendy, chic if she takes care to choose those

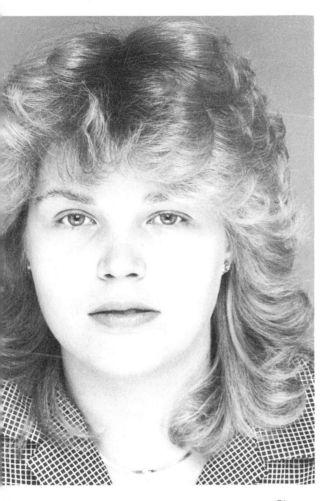

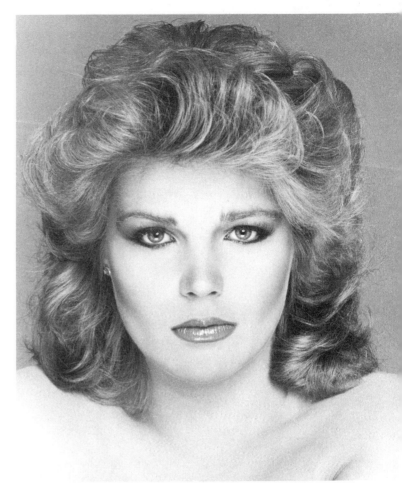

Susan Rogers

A model for Plus Women, one of the first model agencies in New York to feature big, beautiful women, Susan is a perfect example of how contour, color and shadows can make an anonymous round face into nothing less than gorgeous!

---

fashion items that are right for her. The same goes for skin care and makeup, which are just as crucial to her emotional, social and career needs as her closet. And those needs are special and somewhat different from her thinner sister's.

First, Skin Care

Heavy women perspire more than thin women—that's a fact of life. Their body temperature is simply higher. As a result, the pore openings of the body and face tend to become easily clogged with the higher volume of perspiration. Bacteria and fungus infections abound. That is why it's an excellent idea to avoid further clogging those pores with occlusive creams, oils and heavy foundations. It's extremely important to exfoliate often and to be meticulous about giving yourself facials.

Blackheads and pimples are a particular problem for heavy women because of the stepped-up sweat production and gland activity. *Don't squeeze them.* See my skin care cleanliness routine in Chapter 2 for overall preventive measures.

Dilated capillaries, the spidery red lines many big women develop, can be masked with concealer or removed by a medical doctor with electrocautery, which causes the blood to coagulate and the capillaries to turn white.

Avoid facial massage, which breaks down connective tissue, and crash diets—they cause the skin to sag.

TIPS ABOUT DEODORANTS   The heavy woman needs them—you *do* perspire more. If you've been exercising heavily don't jump into a shower immediately upon stopping, because the eccrine sweat glands which release sweat keep working for about fifteen minutes after you've stopped vigorous exercise—so wait that long before a cleansing shower. Don't use an antiperspirant or a deodorant immediately after showering, either. You will be hot and sweaty from the air temperature and the product will be diluted by increased perspiration: wait twenty minutes.

Now, Makeup

Fleshy eyes can be made to look less fleshy and wider by darker shades of eye shadow on the fatty parts and lighter shades on the area under the brows. Cheekbones submerged in fat can be pulled out by contouring cleverly. Jowls and chins can be made to subside and disappear by use of contour.

Unfair, but true: when a skinny mini doesn't tweeze her eyebrows for two weeks and lets her mustache grow, she looks bad. When you do it, you look bad *and* people think "You Slob!" It's unfair, but you have to be more vigilant, take more time, be more careful if you want to dispel the image that fat is unpretty.

FOUNDATION   All foundations that heavy women use should be water- or aloe-based and not oil-based—no matter what the skin type is. That is because of the extra perspiration, and water-based foundations don't melt off the face as quickly as oil-based products do. What's more, there's less of a chance they'll clog your pores. Large women have a more reddish tone to their skins because their adrenaline pumps a little faster, the blood vessels are closer to the surface of the skin and their skin is stretched a little tauter and thinner. They're also subject to broken capillaries which adds ruddiness. Always choose a foundation in a beige tone, a half shade lighter than your complexion, rather than a peach, rose or pink tone. You don't need that extra glow of color.

Big women often have hormone imbalances that can result in facial hair: Dark foundations make the hair and lines on your face more obvious because they *stain* them. Furthermore, many big women have blue in their lips: Make sure you apply the foundation over your lips as well as your face to mask that blue, if you wish your lipstick color to be brighter and clearer.

CONTOURING   Apply, as with everyone, *over* the foundation base, not under it. Shade your entire neck—just paint it out—with contour. It gives a beautiful look and lengthens the neck, as well.

EYES   It's essential that you powder the lids with a translucent powder (or light tone) to prevent the shadow color you choose from being "sweated off." All shadows should be in powder rather than cream form, to prevent them from congealing in the creases.

A darker beige, brown or grey goes on the lid, crease and fleshy overhang that many big women have. *Never* green, blue or any other pastels. The area under the brow should be lightened with beiges, pinks or yellows—never white: white's unnatural.

Use a *liquid* rather than a pencil eyeliner because it won't smudge into fleshy eye folds. Jet black is too harsh; try a dark plum, blue or charcoal.

BROWS   The thinner the brow, the fatter the rest of the face looks. Your brows should be full but cleanly plucked and gently arched up and out to accent your eyes.

Finish with translucent powder to give a matte finish.

*

In another section of this book, I put my distaste for "kitchen cosmetics" on record. But if ever anyone shouldn't fool with yogurt, Crisco, mayonnaise or peaches and cream on her face it's the heavier woman, whose pores clog more easily than a woman with less of a tendency to perspire. Thick, creamy *food* on your face will give you misery.

BLACK BEAUTY AND SKIN CARE

You've been ignored for too long. Either thrust into the "natural" trap because makeup artists didn't know how to enhance your rich and lush skin tones or thrust into the "white" trap because there was nothing else available—you've had makeup problems that would make *anyone* sigh in despair. Even many cosmetic companies supposedly banked towards the black woman have ignored the true needs of the black skin. To all this, I can only say: if you have to, improvise. Never settle for a color which would look fabulous on a natural blond. Never settle for the outlandish and stark oranges and pinks that not-enough-research-money has fi-

nally decided to offer you through the black cosmetic enterprises. Experiment, blend your own if necessary, but make sure your true colors show through and are gloriously pointed up!

The makeup offered, for the most part, to skin darker than olive belongs in the dark ages—and that's history, not color. Black skin care is practically ignored except by an occasional nod in the general direction by writers who want to broaden their readership rather than give genuine help.

Here are some important things to know about the problems of maintenance of black skin.

Donnita George

A jewel selling jewels at Tiffany's:
One day Donnita will be modeling them!

SPECIAL CHARACTERISTICS	SPECIAL SOLUTIONS
DARKENING: Certain body areas tend to become darker than others, including knees, lower buttocks, earlobes, elbows, back of neck and facial areas that receive a kind of daily "rubbing" trauma. If you're in the habit of sitting with your chin in your hand every day, the chin area will take on a darker tone. This "hyperpigmentation" also comes from using strong "peeling" agents like vitamin A gel or solution and 10 percent benzoyl peroxide. Fooling with pimples will do it all the time! Remember: The more attrition you give to your skin, the patchier (darker and sometimes lighter) it will get.	The best tip: Keep your hands away from your face. Whatever you do, don't brush, rub or scrub to lighten any darkening areas. Never use strong peeling agents. Bleaching creams usually make matters worse and Buf-Puf type irritants are to be avoided.
ASHY COLOR: A pale, greyish white color and often a scaliness appears on facial areas and, often, the arms and legs as well. It seems to be particularly prevalent in the wintertime, especially when the home heating is turned up high.	Turn down the heat or get a humidifier: Your skin is getting greyish because it desperately lacks moisture. (A pan of water on the radiator works as well as a humidifier.) Use moisturizers *faithfully,* and I *don't* mean greasing your skin with oil products like Vaseline, baby oil, mineral oil or cocoa butter. That is sure to only make you shiny and block sweat pores (which instigates itching, infection or burning). Another great aid in ash-prevention is cutting down on the strong, drying soaps you may be using.
LIGHTENING: If you hate dark patches you are surely not going to love light ones. But hypopigmentation, the blotchy, almost freckled appearance caused by healing of skin irritations, is a problem for many black women.	Stay away from blemishes! Stop picking, instantly! If it itches, use a cool cloth—don't scratch. Leave surface irritations alone and if you have trouble with healing, you may need a medicated cream (doctor prescribed).
KELOIDS: These are scars of thick, dark, fibrous tissue which may be even larger than the original wound that caused them. Teen-aged girls often get them on earlobes after having their ears pierced, and in the neck, chin and bracelet areas from wearing heavy jewelry. Any time you have skin that's damaged or broken, a keloid may form as it heals. Whites get them also, but hardly at all compared to blacks.	They can be treated most optimally by steroid injections and somewhat less successfully by dry ice and X rays. Again, it is my suggestion that a plastic surgeon be consulted for serious keloid scarring, rather than a dermatologist.

SPECIAL CHARACTERISTICS	SPECIAL SOLUTIONS
FLESH MOLES: Found on many black Americans but rarely in Europeans—they're darker than the normal skin color and raised in little bumps. They come first in the early years and grow in size and number as you age.	If they're not bad, leave them alone: Removal could produce larger keloids. If they're obtrusive, see a plastic surgeon. Creams don't help: They have to be burned off or removed with electrocautery.
CHLOASMA (sometimes called Melasma): Sometimes, especially when your body is in the midst of hormonal changes (as during puberty and pregnancy), a certain darkening of color comes across the center of the face, looking almost like a mask. It can be permanent if you don't do something about it.	Very often, the condition is precipitated by the hormones in birth control pills. You may have to find another method of contraception. If this is the case with you, go see a gynecologist. If it comes during pregnancy, it often disappears slowly after the baby's birth. No cosmetic cream will cure this condition but proper makeup can disguise it. If you suspect you have chloasma, stay out of the sun; also wear a sunscreen lotion containing benzophenone.
VITILIGO: White spots or a loss of pigment sometimes occur and no one knows why. Women with diabetes, thyroid problems and family history of vitiligo seem to be most affected.	My medical friends tell me that a medication called Psoralen used in conjunction with sunlight or ultraviolet light seems to help. My clients have learned to cover up this whitening with a cream foundation.
CREAM DEPILATORIES REACTIONS: Facial hair removers often cause general redness or irritation: If you find this is happening (and black women tend to have loss or gain in pigment with irritation) stop using it!	Waxing is the answer! Be careful with electrolysis which can leave keloid scars. Bleaching creams can permanently bleach your skin as well as facial hairs, so beware also.
POMADE PIMPLES: Although this is not a hairstyling book, facial skin can have problems from black hair styles which require the use of pomades or any heavy hair grease used to make the hair more straight. The grease moves down, via hands and hair, to the forehead where the oil blocks the skin's oil pores and glands. Result? Blemishes, acne—the Pomade Pits!	You're more "in" with an Afro, anyway, but if you really love the straighter hair styles, either straighten chemically or wash your hands very often and keep them away from your face as much as possible. Bangs, saturated with pomade, are disaster for your skin.

If black skin has its pitfalls, it also has its wonders. You can be a sun-child because the melanin content of your skin acts as a filter, letting fewer of those damaging ultraviolet rays through. But everything in moderation—even sun.

You've read that your skin is oilier than Caucasian skin? False! Black women don't have oilier skin than anyone else: it just appears so, because dark surfaces reflect oil and light differently than light surfaces do, and the same amount of oil on Lena Horne looks shinier than it would on Cheryl Tiegs.

Skin Care for the Black Woman

Cleansing cream which contains no water but only oil and solvents is the *worst* thing for your skin. Products like Albolene clean *and* they also, in my opinion, clog and grease. Use only water-based cleansers.

Astringents with alcohol are overly drying and should be avoided like the plague by black women who become ashen with dry skin.

Your skin care and maintenance program should be essentially the same as your white sister's—with one exception. If you are giving yourself two or three exfoliation treatments a week in conjunction with two or three facial masques, only use the exfoliation process for *one* of those facials, because even minor trauma to the black skin can sometimes cause a change in pigmentation. Exfoliating the outer layer of skin *may* be mildly abrasive for your very sensitive skin. Of course, if you have no problems at all with one exfoliation weekly, you can go on to more. If your skin becomes at all blotchy with the exfoliation process, stop it completely—and go on to the masque. It goes without saying that chemical face peels and

dermabrasion of any sort are absolutely out for you!

Makeup

SOME SURPRISING FACTS TO KEEP IN MIND

* Do you know that black skin usually has much blue in it?

* Do you know that many ''filler'' substances in foundations geared for white skin have umber in them? Umber can turn black skin an eerie yellow or even red. Check the labels on each cosmetic product.

* Do you know that dark brown or blackish eye shadows make you look as if you had either hyperpigmentation of the eyelid or a black eye?

* Do you know that you're not the only black woman with practically nonexistent eyelashes? Thinner, shorter, curlier lashes seem to be a racial trademark for many.

* Do you know that great globs of clear gloss on your lips don't make them look smaller but exactly the opposite? Applying lipstick to just the center of your mouth has the same effect.

Although you'll use the same types of products as white women, the colors, techniques and consistencies are often different. Here, broken down into products, are some of the differences that the black woman should consider.

FOUNDATIONS First of all, despite the media hype that pressures you to buy more, more—if you are black and you have a good skin—you need much less foundation. In fact, if your skin is richly colored without blemishes or spotting, you don't need a foundation at all. Now, maybe that's heresy coming from a makeup artist, but if you think about it, white women with tans rarely use foundation. If you have it naturally, revel in your luck. Of course, if your skin is pigmented or acne-troubled, you *will* use a foundation to even out the color—not to give color.

Colors: stay away from the pinks that are greying to you, the orange tints that make you look garish and the beiges that project a lovely shade of green on most black skin. Sometimes, a deep bronze gel is just the thing to make your complexion look more uniform. Janet Langhart, the television reporter, uses an "earthy, ruddy, henna color" in a brand called Indian Earth. Many dark-skinned models often use a foundation with blue undertones. They know they have the same blues in their skin.

POWDER   I've read in many books written by makeup artists that translucent powder turns grey on black skins. It has been my experience that this *rarely* happens. Try it first: If you do notice a whitening effect, try a tinted powder (tinted anywhere from tan to brown). But, do try the translucent first: If it works for you (and I suspect it will), it is far superior to the tinted shades, which only serve to change the color of your carefully chosen foundation.

CONTOUR   The colors you'll use to give your face planes and bones will be rusty brick. Keep these wise words in mind about orange: *it is a color to be used only on fruit. Not faces.*

EYE MAKEUP   Those wonderful doe-brown eyes that most black women have are best complemented *not* by the light pastels— the blues, greens and lavender—but by the *drama* colors—the navies, deep violets, bottle greens.

If you have protruding eyes, certainly *never* use the paler shadows or the pearlized colors. The texture of your eye shadows

should always be *matte,* not glossy. Golds, bronzes, coppers that are artfully blended are usually wonderful on black women but *not* if they have protruding eyes. Remember: flashy light brings out and accentuates; dark subdues.

SPECIAL TIPS

* Model Beverly Johnson puts a touch of black honey lip gloss on the ends of her mascaraed, curled lashes for a truly exciting effect!

* Did you ever try kohl, the Egyptian eye shadow? It works beautifully on some black women.

* Transparent colors were made for you and that's why some of the new gels that add to and highlight the many wonderful colors that make up black skin are so effective. Gels are for eyes as well as faces.

Confused about colors? If your skin is *light brown,* rusts, apricots and seaweed green are great for your eyes. Corals and peaches are wonderful for cheeks and lips. *Medium-dark skin* calls for golds, greys and wines on the eyes; plums, dark reds, roses and deep corals on the cheeks and lips. *Very dark skin* begs for the colors that complement the blues in it, like roses, burgundies, dark blues and copper on the eyes. Cheeks and lips are dynamic with wines, apples, grapes and magentas.

LIP MAKEUP   Too many black women who have very full mouths spend time trying to disguise them and make them smaller. It never works. You can deemphasize in certain ways, but to draw a lip-line a quarter of an inch smaller than your naturally sensual full mouth is unattractive and senseless. Enhance your mouth: use luscious colors and neat outlines. Make the most of your hereditary characteristics instead of trying to fit into a circumscribed mold of beauty.

Colors: Avoid pinks and oranges. The dark burgundies, purples, copper and even, sometimes, lush reds are wonderful for your dusky complexion. Browns look too dark and do nothing for you. If you use a gloss, take a brush and mix it with some color so the application is part gloss, part lipstick—not all gloss. Sometimes the black woman's lower lip will be lighter and pinker than her upper one: Make sure you apply a foundation on your lips before you apply color, so that when the color is applied it will not go on in two different shades. Lips that are very full will look somewhat less full with this coat of foundation. Use a burgundy lip liner, drawing the lip outline *just* inside the outer natural lip-line.

HELLO PREGNANCY: GOODBYE (FOR A WHILE) GREAT SKIN

Thought you'd left adolescent acne behind? Well, along with morning sickness comes that oily, pimply skin that plagued you when you were sixteen. That's just at the beginning of pregnancy. The sebaceous glands speed up oil production in response to hormonal activity. Towards the end, thank goodness, your skin seems to remember you've passed puberty and it never looks better. Keep right up with your skin care program and don't lose heart when it doesn't seem to be working for those first few months. It will. Another story altogether are the moles that seem to appear during the *last* of the nine months. If you can't live with them, they can be easily removed after the baby arrives. Because of hormone changes, scars on the face may become darker. Blotches may also appear. Watch out for those tiny spidery red blood vessels on the face that appear during pregnancy, but that often disappear after the birth of your baby (if they don't, electrocautery can be used to get rid of them quite easily). The mask of pregnancy (chloasma or melasma) is a darkening of pigmentation across the center of the face, also caused by hormonal changes; it almost always disappears after childbirth, even if many other skin pigmentation changes do remain.

Whatever you're noticing, it probably is different from what your skin did before pregnancy. Oily skin now seems dry and flaky and dry skin is going crazy with the greasies. That's par for the course and very normal. It's my advice to stay away from soaps even if you've always used them successfully. Alkaline and medicated soaps can really aggravate the skin problems brought on by pregnancy. Drink lots of water to moisturize, exfoliate religiously, eat a balanced diet and get enough sleep.

SPECIAL TIPS

✳ Coffee, tea and cola drinks seem to aggravate "pregnant" skin.

✳ It's a good idea to avoid direct sunlight as much as possible, say the beauty *and* the medical experts. Use a sunblock with a sun protection factor of 15 as a makeup base instead of a moisturizer, and on top of the sunblock you can use an even heavier-than-usual foundation.

✳ Even if you've always successfully used

products with fragrance added, it's a good idea to temporarily stop. During pregnancy, skin often reacts with irritation to substances it's always been able to tolerate before.

What are those hanging things? During pregnancy, many of my clients report little "skin tags" developing around their necks —fleshy little bits of skin hanging down. These may be removed by a doctor after you've delivered your baby, if they don't disappear all by themselves.

I am so itchy! Don't worry. About a fifth of all pregnant women are also scratching. Bile acids in the skin are building up because the estrogen and progesterone affect the liver and cause it to retain what's normally excreted. This is called cholestasis, say my medical friends, and if it gets really terrible medication can dull the itching.

To sum up, having a baby is an enormous change to the body. Don't be surprised if your skin announces your pregnancy before you do. The good news is that most of the unpleasant changes seem to clear up within three or four months of delivery no matter what you do or don't do.

MAKEUP FOR SPECIAL TIMES

Beauty in the Bed

Who says you can't wear makeup to bed? Well, I did. Very emphatically. There are, however, certain exceptions.

If you're used to curlers and thick layers of cream on the face before sleep, scratch that look when you're entertaining in bed. Also, scratch the foundation-on-the-face look: It will give you grief in the morning in the shape of zits. You *can* gloss your mouth in a soft, berry gel: Not only can that not hurt, it can provide lubrication for your lips, all night. You can, *very lightly,* line the inside of your eyes (the cushy part) with a soft pencil to add luminous depth to your eyes. And you can, *very lightly,* put a coat of mascara on your lashes (anything thick will surely smear). That's it. You never want to put base or blusher or rouge on your face: That will do its dirty work faster than its restorative work. All this is based on the fact that you plan to keep the lights on. Otherwise, why bother? When you're ready to sleep, a quick rinse wouldn't hurt.

Beauty on the Beach

Although it's not traditional, a light coat of foundation is wonderful to wear to the beach. It both blocks the ultraviolet rays (not completely, but enough to take the searing edge off) and gives you your prettiest look. Be sure you choose a waterproof mascara. Lip gloss adds an extra protective sheen to your mouth: Burned lips are not such a unique occurrence, and the dryness and flaking that come *after* a sunburned mouth starts to heal can be enormously aggravating.

Beauty and the Blues

No matter what the reason for a good crying jag, the results are inevitable: puffy eyes, reddened nose, swelling under the eyes. Here then, a fast route to a comeback.

CRYING JAG COMEBACK

1. Take a Coets or cotton ball and gently wash your face clean with a mild cleansing lotion. Tears can be quite irritating to skin.

2. Rinse with cold water: this reduces the superficial swelling.

3. Take an ice cube and gently massage it on the puffy areas around the eye—terrific for swelling. (Even though I am generally opposed to extremes of temperature on the face, in an emergency there's no choice.)

4. Take a minute and lie down with several pillows under your head to encourage water retaining tissues to drain out. A cotton pad dipped in some witch hazel or cooled tea (the cheapest tea has the most tannic acid, which reduces swelling) and placed on each eye will also dissipate redness and swelling.

5. Apply a fresh layer of moisturizer and foundation, blend well, powder.

6. If eyes are still somewhat red, lining the wet ledge of the lower lash-line with a marine or mauve pencil does wonders to make the whites look clearer and brighter, and a drop or two of Murine or another redness-banishing eye-drop can't hurt either.

7. Remembering that darkness hides and light brings out, cover the puffiness under your eye with a soft sable brown or taupe, and use a brighter shade of eye shadow just under the brow to draw attention away from the puffiness. A vibrant shade of lipstick will also draw attention away from the puffiness.

Don't do anything drastic in your melancholy, like hacking away at your hair or changing its color or rushing over to the plastic surgeon to sign up for a nose job.

Beauty for the Blurry-Eyed

The most nervous women are those who have to deal with makeup, especially eye-makeup, and their lenses. Why in the world would anyone who wears contact lenses take them *out* before she applies her makeup? How can she see to get the lip liner on straight if her lenses are in their case? No need to worry about applying eye-makeup with lenses on: You can do everything if you do it slowly and carefully, including the curling of the lashes, the shadows, the mascara. This goes for hard *or* soft lens wearing.

When you wear lenses, it's a good idea to stay away from mascaras which contain fibers that are supposed to thicken and elongate the lashes. What the fibers do, instead, is get in your eye, and *under* your lens, creating an *awful* mess. Lens wearers may be more comfortable with liquid liner as opposed to pencil liner which goes on more evenly, without applying pressure to the lid. The only time you have to take your lenses out is when you *remove* your makeup. Doing a good job here doesn't depend on seeing so brilliantly, and it's better to avoid the possibility of eye irritation with some vagrant colors that end up *in* the eye.

If you wear glasses and not contact lenses, try a special makeup eyeglass-frame available in most eyeglass stores. Each lens folds down on the cheek so you can apply makeup to that eye while looking through the lens that is not folded down.

WISE WORDS FOR EYEGLASS WEARERS

✲ If your makeup is smudged or worn off the area under your eyes where your glasses hit, they are not fitting properly. The weight is causing them to fall forward and rest on your face—it should *not* happen. Bring them to the optician to tighten the shafts so the glasses rest on the bridge of your nose instead of your cheeks.

* A touch of blusher just *above* the brow gives eyes dance and glow.

* Don't pile the eye-makeup on: That won't make the viewer *not* notice your glasses. It also won't do much for your eyes. Blend the shadows in as subtle a way as you would if there were no glasses in front.

* Frames should not be the same shape as your face. Opposites go better: round frames for square faces, square frames to widen narrow or long faces. Pudgy, round faces look fatter in rimless, round frames.

* Coordinate your glasses with your skin tone, eyes or hair: Lens tints should match your skin tone because the wrong color lens can make you look perpetually drained and tired.

* Wear plenty of black mascara to give your eyes the depth that glasses tend to take away: Apply the mascara under and on top of the bottom lashes, as well as the top ones.

* Glasses should follow the natural brow-line: Frames should be level with or slightly above the brow.

* If your skin tone is pink or rosy, cool green, grey and blue lenses and frames will most flatter you. If your skin tone is olive or pale, warm browns, plums, mauves and rusts are for you. Amber frames flatter almost everyone.

* Rhinestones are out. If you wear rhinestones, you must put on a fake beauty mark and a polyester rose in your hair.

* Love the Greta Garbo shades look? If the lenses are grey, green, brown or gold they'll protect the eyes from glaring sun. Blue, pink and yellow lenses may look movie-star-ish, but they don't do a thing for glare protection.

* Minimize puffiness under the eyes by wearing rounder frames with thicker widths instead of frameless or wire-frame jobbies.

* Wear your full array of eye-makeup when you go to buy glasses: Check to see that the lens is large enough to let the color of the shadows come through.

6*

Cosmetic Facial Surgery: How to Avoid the Glazed Ham Look

WE'VE COME FULL CIRCLE. I believe that skin care and makeup can change your life. Literally. I've seen hundreds of women who were frustrated and uneasy about their self-image become positively jubilant and renewed when they learned how to make themselves pretty. Professional and emotional gains are crucial to making a whole woman, but I'm convinced that everything comes easier when you feel you're good looking. But, what happens if absolutely nothing works? I hate to admit it, but sometimes (albeit rarely) makeup and skin care simply don't work out for everyone. There may be something basic about the way you look that just makes you uncomfortable and always has. You take care of your skin health, you make the most of your appearance with flattering, even magical, makeup—and still, absolutely every time you look in the mirror, all you see are those loathed lines. Or that sagging chin. Or that eye-overhang.

When you've tried everything else, and you're still unhappy about your face, there's one thing left to try—it's cosmetic facial surgery. You're worried that . . . people will think you're vain; it will hurt; it won't work.

Cosmetic surgery, once a plaything of the rich and famous, has now become the most popular option of almost anyone who wishes, for aesthetic or economic reasons, to improve her or his appearance. Although such surgery will not remodel your real or imagined personality problems, there's no question that if someone feels she looks better, she will feel better about herself.

What follows are some basic things to consider about the nature of the procedures, which I learned from Dr. Peter Linden, an attending plastic surgeon in several New York City hospitals and the plastic surgeon for Nantucket Island in Massachusetts.

To begin, some wise words.

In our society, like it or not, a premium is placed on looking good and looking youthful. In spite of the fact that aging *should* be associated with maturity and wisdom, aging business people may rightly feel that looking more youthful can help them to achieve more goals. Improving one's facial appearance *may* give one a renewed outlook on possibilities. Thus, the economic aspect to cosmetic surgery cannot be overlooked.

Face-lifts and other cosmetic surgery to provide a more youthful appearance can turn back the clock but they can't stop the ticking. Faces are not static; they always change, the same way your mind should. No operation can permanently prevent an aging appearance. (The good news is that, in five to ten years when the skin shows further signs of attrition, more nips and tucks can be taken.)

All lines and extra skin can never be removed. You would look, as I am fond of saying, like a Glazed Ham. Moreover, a face that looked nineteen on a sixty-year-old body would look decadent. Not pretty at all. The idea is to look the best you possibly can at your own age, which requires giving some respect to the years that have passed. A good plastic surgeon knows the difference between making you look just young and making you look wonderful.

One should never have facial surgery *before* it's needed, in the hope it will forestall problems. It won't. Moreover, cosmetic surgery is not for everyone. I have enormous respect for those who are satisfied with the way they look or who feel there are other, pressing priorities. On the other hand, there are surely busy, thoughtful, intelligent people who opted for cosmetic surgery and these, of course, should never feel guilty or overvain for doing so.

In the end, it's a matter of personal choice and lifestyle. People who are judgmental about other peoples' desire to improve themselves either physically or intellectually are generally very insecure about themselves. I believe that the most satisfied and happy people are those who extract every benefit that modern science and civilized thought offer.

Eyelid Surgery (Blepharoplasty)

One of the most "standard, successful operations," eyelid surgery is designed to rid the eye of extra skin or bagginess in the upper lid, crepiness, fatty deposits in the skin under the eye and other aesthetically correctable results of aging or heredity. Because of excess skin, muscle and fat deposits around the eyelid, people tend to look tired even when they're feeling lively.

Incisions, according to Dr. Linden, are made in existing skin lines in the upper eyelid, and within a millimeter or less under the hair follicles of the lower eyelids. When the scars heal, they are essentially invisible. The operation is done, as is most cosmetic surgery, under local anaesthesia almost exclusively, because there is less bleeding and more opportunity to remove the tissue effectively when the patient can look up or down under the doctor's direction. The post-surgery swelling and black and blue aspect of the eye diminish significantly after two or three days, and the rest of the swelling's disappearance depends on how well the patient follows instructions about using ice compresses. The stitches are removed two or three days after the operation. The fatty deposits don't ever come back, but as aging continues it is entirely possible that the skin around the eyelids may again lose tone and elasticity. Eyelid surgery is often performed long before any other cosmetic surgery because the eyes show attrition first.

Chin and Neck Surgery

Chins can be built up (Marilyn Monroe had it done), or, in a more difficult operation (maybe several), they can also be reduced. That "chinless wonder" or "bulldog" look can throw a whole face off, and certain personality characteristics are wrongly and too often attributed to people with chin abnormalities. People with protruding chins often go through life being thought of as stubborn or domineering and those with receding chins are considered weak or cowardly. Double chins, brought about by yo-yo dieting or aging and a corresponding loss of skin elasticity, can be corrected in a procedure called a lipectomy, generally carried out with an overall face-lift. If the problem is too much chin, a lipectomy removes the excess fat and muscle by means of a small incision made under the chin. If the problem is too little chin, silicone is used to build it up. If you have loose, hanging, turkey wattle skin on your neck, the surgeon can lift and tighten it (usually done in conjunction with a face-lift). Recovery times vary depending on the amount of surgery performed, your own healing propensities and the surgeon's skill, but figure on three or four days in the hospital with stitches being removed in five to seven days for chin and neck surgery combined with a face-lift.

The Face-Lift (Rhytidoplasty)

This is the big one. It's an operation to diminish wrinkling caused predominantly by loose skin and to tighten or remove fatty tissues in the face or neck, which tend to sag as one ages. Sometimes the face does not cooperate and looks far older than one feels or acts. In that case, a face-lift to remove redundant skin and reposition or redrape skin over facial bones may be very satisfying. It *cannot* improve the quality or texture of weather-beaten skin; leathery skin etched with many tiny, wrinkled lines will *not* be magically restored to the velvet, liquidy skin of your teens.

Results of face-lifts vary depending on your age, weight and genes. (If you're overweight in your face, it's a good idea to reduce before surgery for longer-lasting results.) In ideal cases, improvement may last from five

to ten years. Hospitalization traditionally requires from three days to a week, with swelling and discoloration going down in seven to ten days. Scars are usually nested in the hairline and around the ear—away from sight. You will not look like a famous model after a face-lift: You will optimally look like you, only somehow a little smoother, younger, less tired looking. This operation is also usually performed under a local anaesthesia. After a face-lift, it's important to avoid direct exposure to the sun for several months as increased swelling and pigmentation may occur.

Peel It Off?

Well, maybe. The chemical face-peel is a form of chemosurgery which, using different chemicals, actually abrades (wears away) the outer layers of the skin. It's *supposed* to peel off those multiple fine wrinkles you can't lay a finger on in a face-lift, but, according to Dr. Linden, the operation has well-documented problems and complications. It's an actual chemical burn which uses phenol to destroy the epidermis (the top layer of skin) and change the dermis underneath. Wrinkles can appear to be straightened out because their actual cellular construction has been altered. What can also occur is the area that's been "burned" can heal in a different color from the rest of the pigmentation on your face. The skin will have an unpredictable reaction to sun exposure and makeup on the skin will not hold as well because of the difference in skin texture.

A chemical face-peel may remove superficial fine, thin wrinkles, but there may be a price to pay, especially if you have olive pigment in your skin (fair skins react better). Facialists and dermatologists are often "in over their heads'' when they perform chemical face-peels, says plastic surgeon Dr. Linden, and lawyers' offices are full of suits against inexperienced practitioners who have created more problems than patients ever thought possible.

Note: Chemosurgery does *nothing* for deep acne pits and may even make them worse.

Dermabrasion

The idea is the same as a face-peel but the process relies on an actual scraping or planing of the face with a tool instead of a chemical. It's supposed to smooth facial areas that have been pitted by acne scars, but it often does not work unless the scars are small and shallow; deep-pitted acne scars are hardly touched by the process. Again, an unscrupulous or inexperienced technician can plane your face too deeply, so the skin cannot rejuvenate itself. That, my friends, is real trouble, and you can end up looking, I hate to say it, like raw liver. Scarring can occur; so can infections.

While dermabrasion and face-peels can be of use, never, never let anyone near your face who does not have a proven track record with the procedures. And a proven track record does not mean a medical degree alone. Although even superficial surgery should never take place *without* the medical credentials, too many doctors have the delicacy of a sledgehammer when it comes to faces. Interview your doctor closely, check out the work done on other patients and be an informed and articulate self-advocate.

Electrocautery

This is a process wherein an experienced practitioner uses an electric needle to get rid of tiny facial ''spider veins.'' If used prop-

erly, with an extremely light, mild touch, the process works; a heavy touch with the needle is a sure scar builder. And stand forewarned—it can hurt!

The Collagen Connection

Sometimes pitted or deeply scarred skin, displeasing indentations and pockmarks can be plumped out by injecting collagen, the natural protein, into the ''dented'' areas. There is little danger involved, according to Dr. Linden, because collagen is an organic substance normally found in skin. Beware the silicone connection, though. Silicone can also be injected into the skin to build it up, but because silicone is synthetic it can be rejected by the body, float around and possibly lodge in and clog various organs—or it can cause thick scars, discolorations or permanent swellings. Many states ban the procedure and many doctors declare silicone injections are dangerous, even when legally permitted.

Seven Questions Most Often Asked About Cosmetic Surgery

1. *How much does this all cost?*

Prices vary geographically and from doctor to doctor. In New York, before the hospital costs are tacked on, a range of fees for full upper and lower eyelid surgery may run between two and five thousand dollars. A face-lift (not including eyelid surgery) can cost between three and seven thousand dollars. Just because a surgeon is more expensive doesn't mean he or she is better; what your fee should take into consideration is the surgeon's experience, expertise, credentials. Insurance rarely covers cosmetic surgery and the cost of elective surgery (surgery you don't need but choose to have anyway) is usually higher than the surgery you must have for your general physical health.

2. *Does it hurt?*

There is usually relatively little pain, incapacity or discomfort after cosmetic surgery, but it is not a joy either. Be prepared for a moderate amount of annoying aches, pains, numbness, nose-clogging (after nasal surgery, you have to breathe through your mouth for a while), and general crankiness due to temporary discomfort.

Sally Jessy Raphael had eyelid surgery just a few days before she came in to be made up and photographed for this book and you can imagine how small the discomfort was that allowed me to apply eye shadow, foundation, etc. to those same eyes.

3. *Should I have a mini-face-lift?*

The mini-lift, employing a much smaller incision, only accomplishes a fraction of a standard face-lift. Most reputable surgeons advise that a mini-lift gives a mini-result.

4. *What happens if I hate it?*

If you buy makeup, arrive home and decide that it's all wrong—you'd be a fool not to return it. It's not as easy with surgery where the general rule is ''no refunds, no exchanges.'' While it is technically possible to redo some surgery that is considered disastrous by the patient, it's a terrible idea to treat a face as a guinea pig, changing, experimenting, redoing original results. There's just so much trauma that skin and bones will take without looking artificial and—not pretty. Be sure you want and need cosmetic surgery before you lie down for the first operation and make sure that the doctor you choose is the very best person you can find. Remember, this is your *face*—not any old molar or hair style.

5. *Is there any other procedure besides dermabrasion or chemical face-peel to diminish wrinkles or acne scars?*

Yes, says Dr. Linden. A skilled plastic surgeon can surgically *shave* a wrinkle down and get results, with the precision involved in going for each individual line, that can't be achieved with either a peel or a dermabrasion. The fine lines above the lip into which lipstick bleeds are particularly helped by the shaving process. Acne scars, in the more severe cases, can often be helped with a skin grafting technique.

6. *I've heard a lot about those new acupuncture face-lifts and massage or laser surgery techniques to improve sagging skin. Is there anything to them?*

Absolutely not. There are dozens of tiny face muscles. Even if you increased the diameter of each one *four to ten times* by facial exercise, needle or laser trauma, you could never make enough of a difference in volume to have any true, visible results. These shortcuts to face-lifts can sometimes relax the face so it looks more rested temporarily, but no true, restorative results are ever, ever seen.

7. *What are the risks of cosmetic surgery?*

They are minimal and rare when done by an accomplished physician. Any operation may have potential problems such as infection or severe bleeding or reactions to anaesthesia, but cosmetic surgery is traditionally easy and straightforward with rare problems.

The very best way to get the very best results from cosmetic surgery is to question your doctor very closely. If the plastic surgeon you choose seems to be in a hurry, makes fun of or is sarcastic about your questions, doesn't seem to know answers or to be *willing* to answer—get out while the getting's good. Better to have a lot of wrinkles than a botched job, or a doctor who makes you miserable.

To sum up: with cosmetic surgery, you makes your choices and you takes your chances that the "new you" will make you prettier, happier and more confident than the old you. Here are a half-dozen cautions that Dr. Linden and other reputable plastic surgeons offer.

＊ Cosmetic surgery is not a supermarket. You cannot bring in pictures of one model's nose and another's chin or skin and say "I want one of those, one of those and one of those . . ." The changes that are made on your face must be in harmony with the rest of the face.

＊ Patients often look at their lives in different ways after surgery, but surgery can't drastically change deep unhappiness or dissatisfaction. "But," says Dr. Linden, "if a person's psychological problems are directly related to a true disharmony in her face, why shouldn't she have it corrected and put her energies elsewhere?" The rule of thumb is: have it done if you need it and want it; don't have it done if you don't need it—even if you want it.

＊ Too young, too old for cosmetic surgery? It's a wrong question to ask, most of the time. Once full, normal growth of the features has been attained, age has little to do with cosmetic surgery, and general health and need has everything to do with it.

＊ Choose your physician as carefully (maybe more carefully) as you do your mate.

Look for: board certification and specialty training; affiliations with good hospitals or clinics; experience in cosmetic surgery, particularly in the specific area in which you're interested.

Ask for: photographs of pre- and post-operation of other patients (if *every* nose job looks like Debbie Boone's nose, the doctor is not an artist); recommendations from other patients and from your family doctor.

＊ Always get a second opinion, as you should with any surgery.
＊ Don't become a cosmetic surgery fanatic; if you find yourself thinking about a fourth face-lift, perhaps you ought to see a psychiatrist instead of getting a lift.

The Last Word

Before you make a decision on cosmetic surgery, consider this one thought, very carefully: Are you absolutely sure that judicious application of makeup won't solve most of your problems?

Point One: Sometimes makeup can be a terrific instant face-lift and it costs you nothing in comparison with the serious kind of face-lift.

Point Two: Are you really sure that the thing you want to change so much, the largish nose or the slightly asymmetrical feature, isn't the precise thing that makes you so uniquely *you,* so fascinating, so extraordinary?

Once you've had the surgery, you can never get that nose with the aquiline tilt back and you will look just like one of the crowd.

Epilogue

SO THERE YOU ARE: It's not so tough to look terrific, is it? The thing that most saddens me are the excuses I hear:

"I haven't the time."
"I'm not vain about appearances."
"Character counts more than face."

Oh, sure. To me, all the above spells laziness or insecurity.

Women have come far in terms of their own health and expectations. What was once inappropriate is now expected. They're exercising. Only yesterday, they settled for gentle, ineffectual stretches. Today they know that being in shape means *moving*, breathing hard, even, God forbid, sweating—an activity that was previously reserved for he-men. They're climbing those corporate ladders. Yesterday they settled for home and hearth: today they can choose to be anyone they wish. They're claiming prettiness. Yesterday, if they were born pimpled or long-nosed or fleshy-faced, they settled for it because only "street women" wore makeup. Today they know they can look gorgeous, interesting or sexy and also be as *nice* as they truly are.

Skin care and makeup is just an extension of feeling fit, of being all you can be.

It's an affirmation of self. If you have taken the time to make an about-face when it applies to

* health,
* success,
* creating a finer, more whole you . . .

then it stands to reason you will care About Face!

✳ *Index*

Acne, 45
  foods which aggravate, 51
  treatments to avoid, 39
  vitamin A for, 46
Acupuncture face-lifts, 151
Afta Cleaning Fluid, 77
Aging, 42–43
  See also Older women
Air pollution, 42–43
Allergies, 53–54
  to cosmetics, 58
Aloe, 17, 36, 37
Apricots, 24
Aramis, 16, 20
Arden, Elizabeth
  Active Day Protecting Mois-
    ture-Cream, 127
  Bye-Lines, 35
  Moisture Action, 34
  translucent powder, 63
Arpel, Adrien, 24
Astringents, 141
Avocados, 24
Avon, 18

B vitamins, 46, 49
Barbiturates, 49
Beach, makeup to wear to, 144
Beauty "doctors," 22
Bed, makeup to wear in, 144
Bergen, Polly, 17
Beverly Hills Diet, 25

Bialick, Lee, 116
Biba's contour powder, 64
Big women, 134–37
  makeup for, 136–37
  skin care for, 135–36
Black women, 137–43
  makeup for, 141–43
  products marketed to, 20
  skin care for, 141
  soaps to be avoided by, 18
  special characteristics of,
    139–40
Blackheads, 31–32, 136
  emergency fixes for, 39
Blending, 77, 80, 134
Blepharoplasty, 148
Blusher, 57
  application of, 65
  mistakes with, 80
  for older women, 133–34
Bonne Bell products, 19
Borghese, 20
  Lumina, 60, 65
Brasivol Lathering Scrub
    Cleanser, 127
Brinkley, Christie, 44, 103
Bronzers, 80
Brow powder, 57
  application of, 65
  for older women, 133
Brows
  of big women, 137
  bleaching, 74

  overemphasis of, 78–79
  shaping, 93
  tweezing, 74–75
Bruce, Shelley, 117

Camomile, 36–37
Capillaries, broken, 53
Carbona Cleaning Fluid, 77
Carmen (model), 130
Casual chic, 100
Chanel
  Démaquillant Doux Cleanser,
    34
  eye crayon, 67
  lipstick, 68
  Teint Naturel Liquid, 60
  translucent powder, 62
Charlie products, 20
Chattem Laboratories Mudd
    Super Cleansing Treat-
    ment, 37
Cheap products, 27–29
Cheekbones
  emphasizing, 107–8
  See also Facial bones
Chemical face-peel, 149–50
Chin
  cosmetic surgery on, 148–49
  makeup to improve, 76–77,
    111–12
Chloasma, 140
Cholesterol, 50, 130

Citric acid, 51
"Civilian doctors," 22–23
Clarins eye cream, 35
Cleansers, 33–34
    for black women, 141
    for teenagers, 126, 128
    used before applying
      makeup, 58–59
Clinique, 18, 20, 26, 29
    Balanced Base, 60
    Clarifying Lotion 2, 34, 127
    Dramatically Different
      Moisturing Lotion, 34
    7th-day Scrub Cream, 26
    Very Emollient Cream, 34
Cold weather, 42–43
Collagen, 36, 37
    injections of, 150
Color strategies, 93–97
    for black women, 142, 143
    for older women, 133–34
Color wash, 134
Concealer
    application of, 62
    mistakes with, 79
    for older women, 132
    tips and tricks with, 77
Contact lenses, 145
Contour powder, 57
    application of, 64
    for big women, 136
    for black women, 142
Contraceptives, 48
Cooper, Marilyn, 87
Cosmetic surgery, 147–52
Cream rouge, 57
    application of, 65
    for older women, 134
Crying jag, repairing damage
    after, 144–45

Dated makeup styles, 78
Denney, Frances, lipstick, 68
Deodorant soaps, 19
Deodorants, 136
Department store salespeople,
    18
DeRibere, Lisa, 122

Dermabrasion, 150
Dermal-feeder moisturizer, 59
Dermatologists, 21–22, 48–49
Diet, 25–26
    effects on skin of, 42–43,
      50–51
DiGennaro, Gloria, 86
Dior, Christian, 20–21
Dipilatories, 140
Doak Pharmacal Formula 405
    Light Textured Moisturizer,
      34
Doe eyes, 79
Do-everything products, 19
Drinking Man's Diet, 25
Dry skin, 41
    checkpoint changes for, 43
Ducat, Lee, 131

Eat All You Want Diet, 25
Eczema, 45
Eggs, 24
Ejection, 36–38
Electrocautery, 150
Elliott, Allison, 111
Erace, 79
Erno Laszlo Institute, 17
Estrogen, 26
Etherea, 20
Evening chic, 102–3
Exercise, 45
Exfoliation, 35–36
    for black women, 141
    for older women, 130
    for teenagers, 127
Experts, 21–23
Eye cream, 35
    for older women, 132
    for teenagers, 127
Eye shadows
    application of, 65–66
    for big women, 137
    for black women, 142
    color combos for, 97
    number needed, 57
    for older women, 133, 134
    for teenagers, 128
    tips and tricks with, 74

Eyelash curler, 58
    for older women, 133
    use of, 75
Eyelid surgery, 148
Eyeliner, 57
    application of, 67
    for big women, 137
    for older women, 133
    for teenagers, 128
    tips and tricks with, 74
Eyes, 83–87
    close set, 84
    hooded, 86–87
    makeup to improve, 106
    Oriental, 86
    protruding, 85
    small, 85
    wide set, 84

Face peels, 149–50
Face-lift, 149
Facial bones
    bringing out, 90
    makeup to improve, 107
    prominent, 91
Facial exercises, 25
Facial hair, 51–52, 136
Facials, 37–38, 40
    for teenagers, 127
False eyelashes, 75
Fashion designers, 22
Fatigue, 48
Ferrare, Christina, 44
Food and Drug Administration,
    free booklets from, 78
Foundation, 57
    application of, 60–61
    for big women, 136
    for black women, 141–42
    for older women, 132
    for teenagers, 128
    tips and tricks with, 77
"Free" merchandise, 16–17
Freshener, 34, 59
    for teenagers, 126
Fritsch, Sherry, 107
Frosteds, 134

Gandhi, Nila, 89
George, Donnita, 138
Glasses, 145–46
Glycerine, 25
Goodwin, Jan, 118
Gray, Dorothy, Cleansing
    Grains, 127
Greenfield, Debra, 112
Gross, Susan, 115

Hair, facial, 51–52, 136
Hairdressers, 22
Halston eye shadow, 66
Health store products, 25
Henderson, Heather, 117
Herpes, 27
Hirsch, Mildred, 116
Hormones, 26
Hubbard, Elizabeth, 113

Ice Cream Diet, 25
Ilona of Hungary, 17
Impressions, creating various,
    98–99
Isotretinoin, 46

Jawlines, makeup to improve,
    111–12
Johnson, Beverly, 142
Jordan, Michelle, 117

Keloids, 139
Kitchen cosmetics, 24–25
Klausner, Terri, 88
Klisar Skin Care Center, 17
Kohl, 142
K2r Spot-lifter, 77

Lactic acid, 51
Lancôme, 16
    Bienfait-Démaquillant, 36
    Galatée Milky Creme
        Cleanser, 34
    Maquiriche CremePowder
        EyeColour, 66
    mascara, 67
    translucent powder, 62
Lanolin, 25
Laser surgery, 151

Lash tricks, 75
Last Chance Diet, 25
Laszlo, Erno, 17
Lauder, Estée, 16, 18, 20, 26, 29
    brow powder, 65
    Pressed Eyelid Shadow, 66
    Re-Nutriv, 34
    Swiss Age-Controlling
        Cream, 26
Lauren, Ralph, 16, 20
Lemons, 24–25
Lewis, Marcia, 90
Lighting, 82–83
    for older women, 130, 132
Linden, Peter, 25, 147–52
Lip-color brush, 58
Lip gloss
    application of, 68
    mistakes with, 80
    number needed, 57
    tips and tricks with, 76
Lip liner, 57
    application of, 68
    for black women, 142–43
    mistakes with, 79–80
    for older women, 133
    tips and tricks with, 75–76
Lipson, Carol, 113
Lipstick
    application of, 68
    for black women, 142–43
    mistakes with, 79
    number needed, 57
    for older women, 133, 134
    tips and tricks with, 75
Little, Rich, 106
Liver spots, 132
Lock, Judy, 76
Loren, Sophia, 129

McGovern, Maureen, 56, 116
Mackay, Lizbeth, 114
Makeup practitioners, 22
Malic acid, 51
Markoff, Alexandra de
    blusher, 65
    eye shadows, 66
Mary Kay, 18

Mascara, 58
    application of, 67
    clumping of, 80
    for older women, 133, 134
    removal of, 34
    for teenagers, 128
    tips and tricks with, 75
Masques, 36–38
    for teenagers, 127
Massage, 25, 151
Mayo Clinic Diet, 25
Medical doctors, 21–22
Medicated soaps, 18
Melasma, 48, 140
Menstruation, 46–47
Michaels, Marilyn, 106
Mini-face-lift, 151
"Miracle" creams, 17
Moisturizer, 34–35, 58, 77
    applied under makeup, 59
    for older women, 130
    for teenagers, 126–28
Moisturizing soap, 18
Moles, 53, 140
Monteil, Germaine, 18, 26
    Super Moist Line-Stop Creme
        Concentrate, 26
Moon Drops, 20
Mouth, makeup to improve, 110
Murine, 145

"Natural" products, 24, 25
Necklines
    cosmetic surgery on, 149
    of older women, 133
Neutrogena, 124
New England Journal of Medicine, 46
New York Clinique de Beauté,
    17
Newman, Phyllis, 115
Normal skin, 41
    checkpoint changes for, 43
Noses, 88–89
    hooked, 89
    makeup to improve, 109
    too short, 89
    wide, 88
Noxzema Complexion Lotion, 19

Office chic, 100
Oily skin, 41
    checkpoint changes for, 42
Older women, 129–34
    makeup for, 132–34
    products marketed to, 20
    skin care for, 129–30
Olive skin, 96
On Stage concealer, 62
Onassis, Jackie, 84
Oral contraceptives, 48
Overpriced products, 20–21

Pan Stick, 79
Peaches, 24
Perfumed soaps, 19
Perspiration, 52–53
Perutz, Katherine, 20
Pfifer, Darcy, 109
pH balance, 27
Phillips, Susan, 69–73
pHISODERM, 126
Pierce, Nina, 115
Pietro, Stephan, 17
Pill, the, 48
Pimples, 31–32, 136
    pomade as cause of, 140
    See also Acne
Pineapples, 25
Placenta masques and extracts,
    26
PMS (premenstrual syndrome),
    46
Polyunsaturated oils, 130
Powder
    colored, 79
    See also Translucent powder
Pregnancy, 42–43, 143–44
Prescriptives, 20
Progesterone, 26
Progrès Plus Creme Anti-Rides,
    35
Psoriasis, 45

Q-Tips, 58

Raccoon eyes, 79
Raphael, Sally Jessy, 108, 151
Reinking, Ann, 113
Relaxation techniques, 45–46
Resorcinol, 18
Retinoic acid, 46
Revlon, 16, 18–20
    Eterna '27', 35
    See also Ultima II
Rhytidoplasty, 149
Rockefeller Diet, 25
Rogers, Susan, 135
Rosacea, 53
Roth, Eda, 81
Rouge
    mistakes with, 80
    See also Cream rouge
Rubenstein, Helena, Eye Cream
    Special, 19
Ruddy skin, 95

Sable brushes, 58
Saint Laurent, Yves, 68
Sallow skin, 94
Salt, 51
Scarsdale Diet, 25
Sensitive skin, 53–54
Sex, 45
Shadow seal, 57
    application of, 65
Sharp, Molly, 100–103
Shelley, Carole, 92
Shields, Brooke, 83, 93
Shine, 79
Shiseido, 37
    moisturizer, 127
Shrimpton, Jean, 79
Silicone injections, 150
Singer, Dominique, 114
Skin, makeup to improve,
    118–19
Skin care practitioners, 22
Skin color, 93–96
Skin type, 40–41
Soaps, 32
    special, 18–19
Southampton Diet, 25

Staining, 77
Stansbury, Hope, 119
Starch Blockers' Diet, 25
Steadying your hand, 77
Steam heat, 43
Steinem, Gloria, 55
Stendahl, 26
Steroids, 49
Stiefel Laboratories, 127
Strawberries, 25
Stress, 45, 48
    during menstruation, 46, 47
    of traveling, 48
Sugar, 51
Sun, 49–50
    overdoses of, 42–43
Sylva, Livia, 17
"Systems," 17–18

Teasdale, Sara, 15
Teenagers, 123–28
    daily cleansing schedule for,
        126–27
    dermatologists and, 22
    makeup for, 128
    products marketed to, 19, 20
    weekly maintenance schedule
        for, 127
Terezakis, Nia K., 36
Tiegs, Cheryl, 103
Touch-ups, 100
Translucent powder, 57
    application of, 62
    for black women, 142
    for teenagers, 128
Tulane Medical School, 36
Turnbull, Stefanie, 110
Tweezers, 58
Twiggy, 79

Ultima II
    CHR, 35
    eye shadows, 66
    lipstick, 68
Ultraviolet treatments, 39

Vacations, skin problems during, 47–48
Valmy, Christine, 17, 20
Valtone Eye and Neck Creme, 20
Van Hamel, Martine, 114
Vanderbilt, Gloria, 16
Vitamin A, 46
Vitamin E, 46
    for older women, 130

Vitiligo, 140
Von Furstenberg, Diane, 68

Warts, 53
Water, 44
Waxing, 52
Weissler, Francie, 91, 125
Weissler, Sheila, 91
Whiteheads, 31–32
Wind, 42–43

Winthrop Laboratories, 126
Wrinkle creams, 26

X-ray therapy, 39

Yogurt, 25

Zits, 31–32

✳ *About the Authors*

JEFFREY BRUCE, despite his relative youth, is considered by those in the know to be one of the finest makeup and skin care experts in the country. His clients include the world's most famous and admired women as well as thousands who have come to him, attracted by his irreverent and honest wit, through television and radio appearances. Bruce's early apprentice work took him behind the scenes at Estēe Lauder, Revlon, Givenchy and the fabled Kenneth where he not only developed his unique talents, but learned enough "secrets" to expose the myths, lies and extravagances of the business he loves. He's a breath of fresh air in the beauty industry, and his clarity and sensible approaches to great skin and cosmetics have made him one of the highest paid artists in the world. He deserves it.

SHERRY SUIB COHEN has written on beauty and other disparate subjects for almost every major magazine in the country. She's the author of five major books which range in topic from Cristina Ferrare to diabetes to parental relationships to health, success and good looks for women.

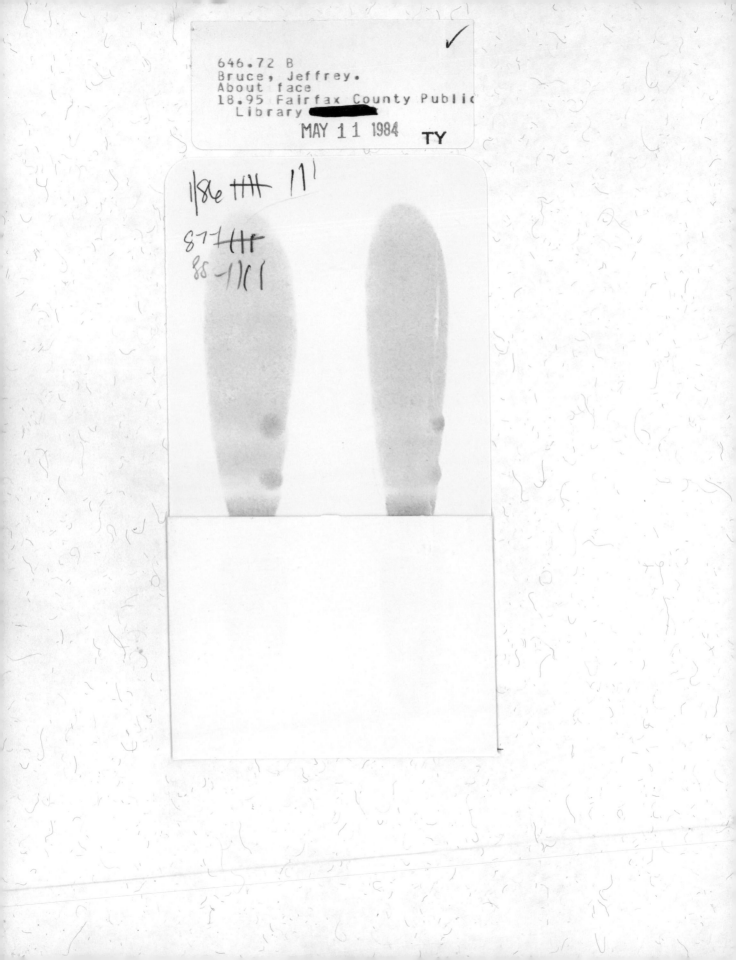